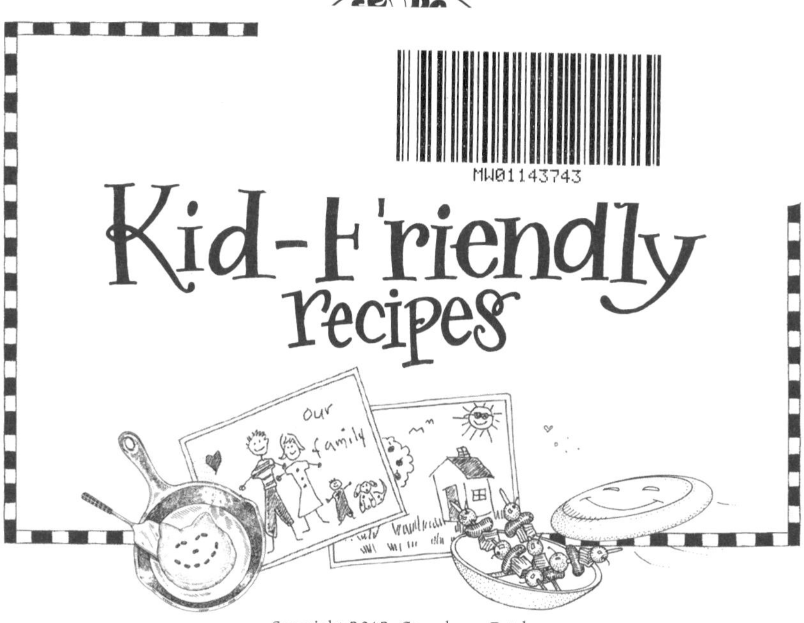




First Printing, March, 2012

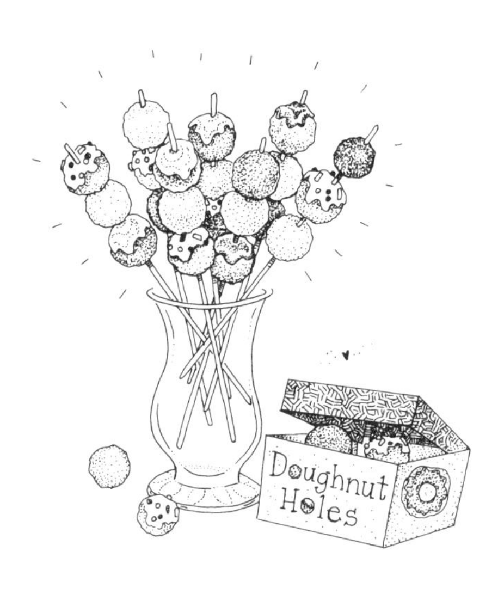


A fun centerpiece for the breakfast table! Thread doughnut holes on long wooden skewers and arrange in a vase for easy serving. Yum!

## Breakfast Banana Split

*Makes one serving*

1 banana
1/2 c. favorite crunchy cereal, divided
1/2 c. fruit-flavored yogurt
1/4 c. blueberries or strawberries, sliced
1/4 c. pineapple chunks, drained
maraschino cherries (optional)

Peel banana and cut down the middle lengthwise with a butter knife. Place banana in a cereal bowl or a banana split dish. Sprinkle half the cereal over the banana. Spoon yogurt over the banana and cereal. Add the rest of the cereal and fruit on top. Add cherries, if you like.

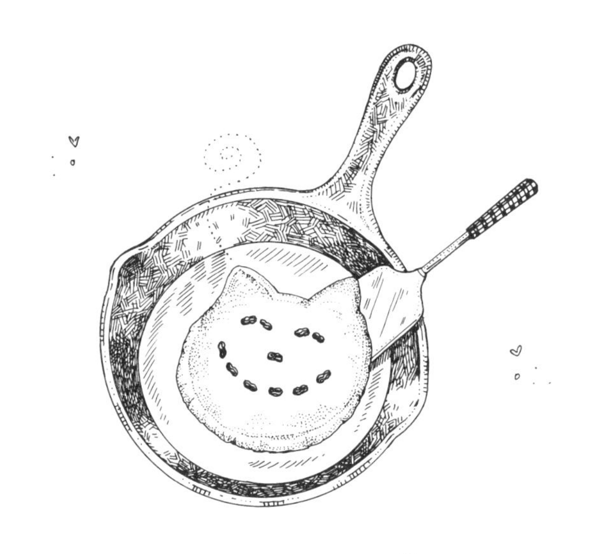

No time for a leisurely breakfast? Try breakfast for dinner...it's sure to become a family favorite!

## Breakfast Pizza

*Makes 6 servings*

8-oz. tube refrigerated crescent rolls
1 lb. ground sausage, browned and drained
1 c. frozen diced potatoes, thawed
1 c. shredded Cheddar cheese
5 eggs
1/4 c. milk
1/2 t. salt
1/8 t. pepper
2 T. grated Parmesan cheese

Separate rolls into 8 triangles. Arrange rolls with points toward the center in an ungreased 12" pizza pan. Press over bottom and up sides to form crust; seal perforations. Spoon browned sausage over crust. Sprinkle with potatoes; top with Cheddar cheese. Set aside. In a bowl, beat together eggs, milk, salt and pepper. Pour over crust. Sprinkle Parmesan cheese over the top. Bake at 375 degrees for 25 to 30 minutes. Cut into wedges to serve.

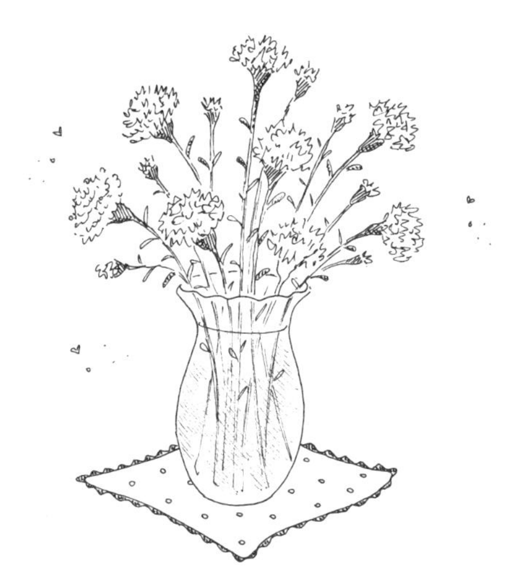

Make white flowers magically turn red, yellow or green! Drop a little food coloring into the water and plain white carnations or Queen Anne's lace will gradually absorb the color. Fun for kids to watch!

## Muffin Doughnuts

*Makes one dozen*

2 c. all-purpose flour
1/2 t. salt
1 T. baking powder
1/2 t. nutmeg
1/2 c. plus 1/2 t. butter, divided
1-1/2 c. sugar, divided
1 egg, beaten
3/4 c. milk
3/4 c. semi-sweet chocolate chips
1/2 c. chopped pecans
2 t. cinnamon

Combine flour, salt, baking powder, nutmeg, 1/2 teaspoon margarine, 1/2 cup sugar, egg and milk. Fold in chocolate chips and pecans. Fill greased muffin cups 2/3 full. Bake at 350 degrees for 20 minutes. Remove immediately from pan. Melt the remaining butter; roll muffins in butter. Combine remaining sugar and cinnamon; roll muffins in mixture.

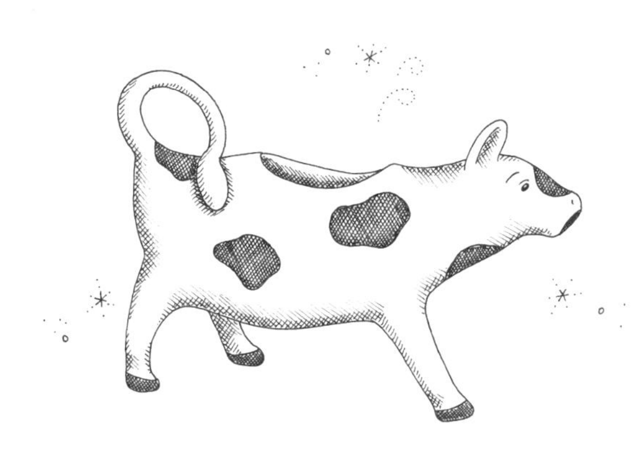

A touch of whimsy...use Grandma's old cow-shaped pitcher to serve milk or cream for breakfast cereal and oatmeal.

## Fantastic Stuffed French Toast

*Serves 6*

5 eggs, beaten
2/3 c. whipping cream
2 t. cinnamon
2 8-oz. pkgs. cream cheese, softened
1 t. vanilla extract
2 loaves Vienna bread, sliced into 3-inch thick slices
12-oz. jar apricot preserves
1/2 c. orange, banana & strawberry juice blend

Whisk together eggs, cream and cinnamon; set aside. Beat cream cheese and vanilla with an electric mixer. Set aside. Slice 3/4 of the way into one edge of each bread slice, creating a pocket. Spoon some of the cream cheese mixture into each bread pocket. Dip slices into egg mixture on both sides. On a griddle over medium heat sprayed with non-stick vegetable spray, cook until golden on both sides. Meanwhile, mix preserves and juice in a small saucepan; simmer over medium heat until slightly thickened. Spoon warm preserves mixture over slices of French toast.

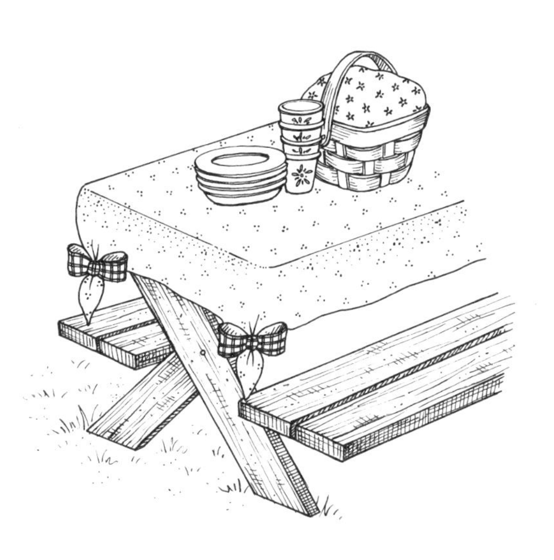

Take breakfast outdoors! Spread a quilt on the picnic table and enjoy the cool morning air.

## Yummy Carrot-Raisin Muffins

*Makes one dozen*

18-oz. pkg. carrot cake mix
15-oz. can pumpkin
1/3 c. golden raisins

Mix dry cake mix and pumpkin together to make a very thick batter. Add raisins and mix well. Fill paper-lined muffin cups 2/3 full. Bake at 400 degrees for 20 minutes, or until muffins test done.

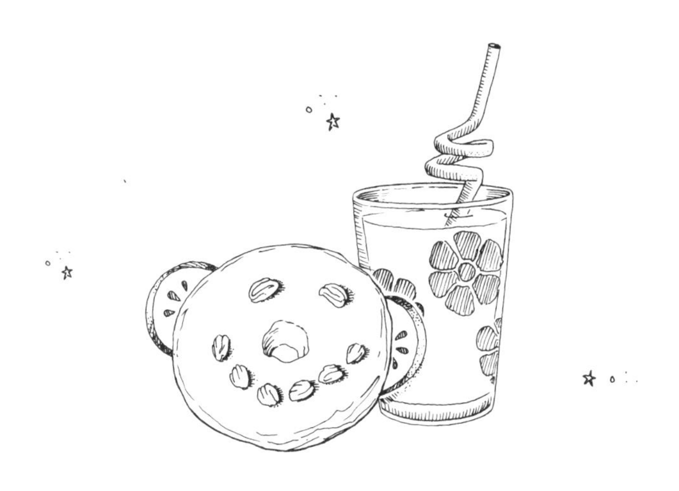

Make breakfast fun! Cut the centers from slices of toast with a cookie cutter, serve milk or juice with twisty straws and put smiley faces on bagels using raisins and cream cheese.

## Good Morning Monkey Bread *Makes 1-1/2 dozen rolls*

18 frozen white dinner rolls
3/4 c. sugar
3/4 c. brown sugar, packed
3-1/2 oz. pkg. cook & serve butterscotch pudding mix
3 to 4 t. cinnamon
1/2 c. butter, sliced
Optional: 1/2 c. chopped pecans

Scatter frozen rolls in a Bundt® pan that has been sprayed with non-stick vegetable spray. Rolls will expand, so take care not to overfill pan. Set aside. In a separate bowl, mix sugars, dry pudding mix and cinnamon together. Sprinkle mixture on top of frozen rolls; dot with butter. Cover pan with a tea towel; let rise overnight. In the morning, uncover and bake at 350 degrees for 30 to 45 minutes. Remove from oven and let stand 15 to 20 minutes. Turn pan over onto a serving tray; spoon warm syrup from pan over bread.

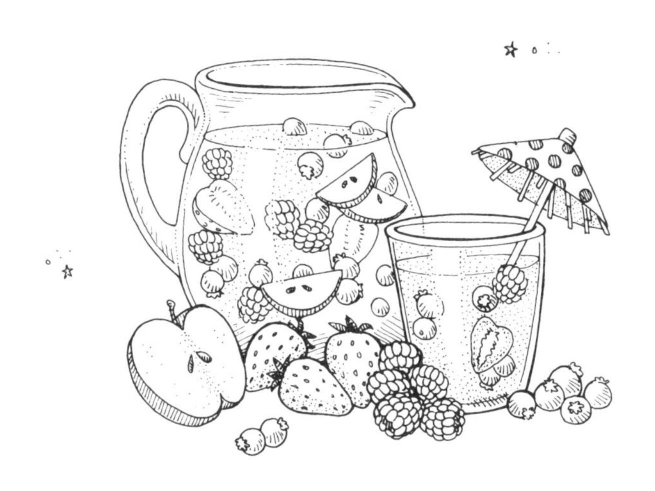

To add a splash of color to breakfast juices, freeze strawberry slices or blueberries in ice cubes. Toss several into glasses of juice right before serving.

# Jumbo Quiche Muffins

*Makes 10 muffins*

16.3-oz. tube refrigerated flaky buttermilk biscuits
1/2 c. cream cheese, softened
4 eggs, beaten
1/4 t. seasoned salt
1/4 t. pepper
6 slices bacon, crisply cooked and crumbled
1/2 c. shredded Cheddar cheese

Place each biscuit into a greased jumbo muffin cup; press to form a well. Combine cream cheese, eggs, salt and pepper. Spoon 2 tablespoons egg mixture into each biscuit well; sprinkle with bacon and top with cheese. Bake at 375 degrees for 15 minutes.

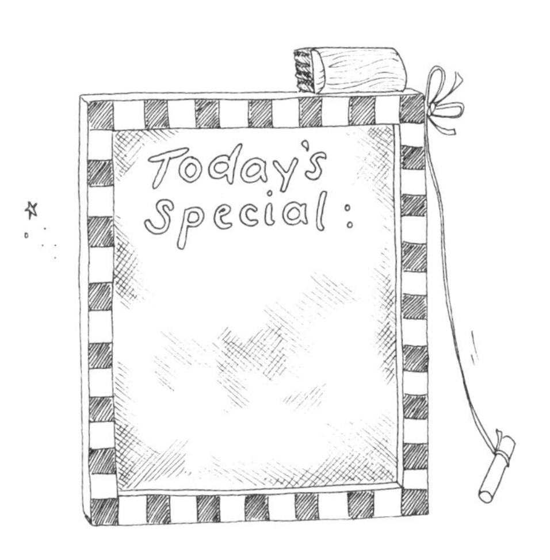


Turn cast-off cabinet doors, a salvaged mirror or old window into a handy kitchen blackboard. Coat any flat surface with chalkboard paint; let dry, then recoat. A lighthearted way to let everyone know what's for dinner!

## ***Berry Bog Oatmeal***

*Serves 4*

1 c. steel-cut oats, uncooked
1 c. sweetened, dried cranberries
1 c. chopped dates
4 c. water
1/2 c. half-and-half
2 T. honey

Combine oats, cranberries, dates and water in a greased slow cooker. Cover and cook on low setting for 6 to 8 hours. Stir in half-and-half and honey; warm through.

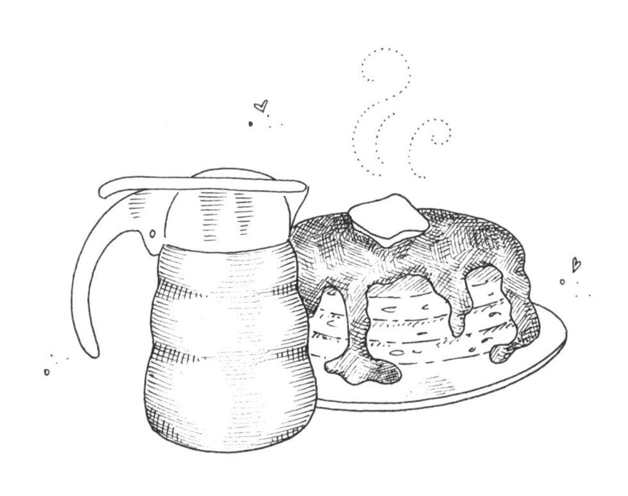

Here's a helpful hint for young chefs...use a washable marker to mark a line on a glass measuring cup, and they'll know just how much to pour.

## Go Bananas Pancakes

*Serves 4*

2 eggs
2 T. sugar
1-1/4 c. all-purpose flour
1 t. baking powder
2-1/2 c. bananas, mashed

Blend eggs and sugar together; mix in flour, baking powder and bananas with a fork. Pour by 1/4 cupfuls onto a hot, buttered griddle; cook until bubbles form along the edges. Flip and cook until golden on the other side.

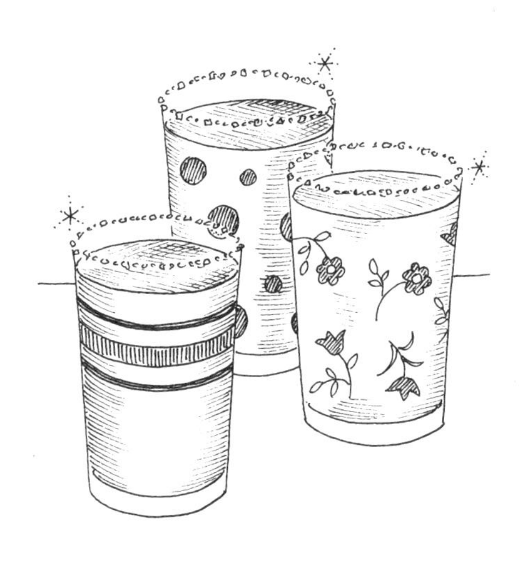

Make juice glasses sparkle! Dip the rims in water and roll in coarse sugar before filling with orange juice.

## Breakfast Apple Sandwiches

*Makes 16 sandwiches*

16.3-oz. tube refrigerated jumbo biscuits
8-oz. pkg. shredded Cheddar cheese, divided
2 apples, cored and sliced into 16 rings
2 T. cinnamon
1/4 c. brown sugar, packed
1/4 c. butter, melted

Split biscuits. Lay each biscuit half on an ungreased baking sheet. Sprinkle about 2 tablespoons of cheese on each biscuit. Top with an apple slice. In a bowl, mix together cinnamon and brown sugar. Spoon some cinnamon-sugar on top of each apple slice. Top with a small amount of butter. Bake, uncovered, at 400 degrees for 15 to 20 minutes, until golden.

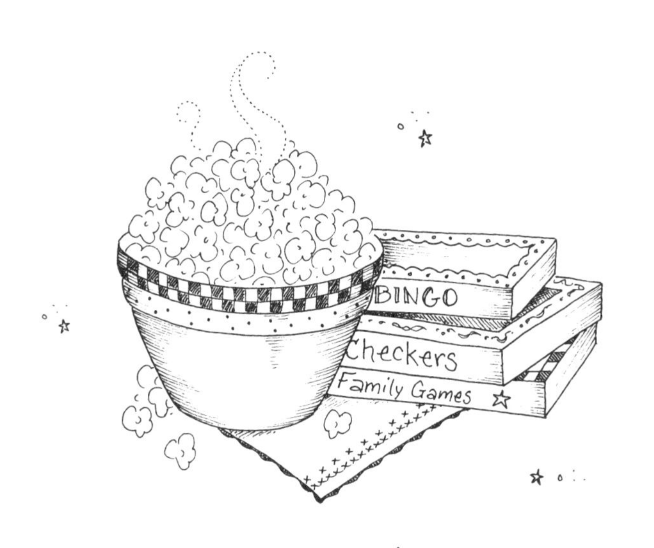


Make tonight a family game night! Get out all your favorite board games and play to your heart's content. Small prizes for winners and bowls of munchies are a must!

## Triple-Take Grilled Cheese

*Makes 4 sandwiches*

1 T. oil
8 slices sourdough bread
1/4 c. butter, softened and divided
4 slices white American cheese
4 slices Muenster cheese
1/4 c. shredded sharp Cheddar cheese
Optional: 4 slices red onion, 4 slices tomato, 1/4 c. chopped fresh basil

Heat oil in a skillet over medium heat. Spread 2 bread slices with one tablespoon butter; place one slice butter-side down on skillet. Layer one slice American, one slice Muenster and 2 tablespoons Cheddar cheese on bread. If desired, top with an onion slice, a tomato slice and one tablespoon basil. Butter another slice of bread; add to sandwich in skillet. Reduce heat to medium-low. Cook until golden on one side, about 3 to 5 minutes; flip and cook until golden on the other side. Repeat with remaining ingredients.

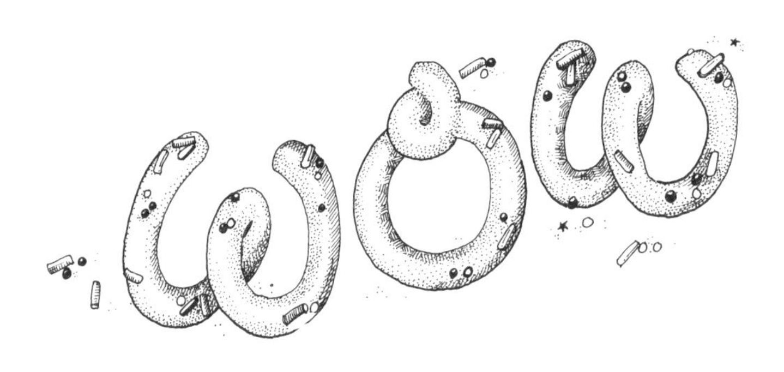

Can you spell YUM? A package of refrigerated bread sticks presents all kinds of alphabet fun... just shape the dough into letters before baking! Sprinkle with cheese, or cinnamon-sugar for a sweet treat.

## Chicken-Tortilla Soup

*Serves 6*

14-1/2 oz. can chicken broth
10-3/4 oz. can cream of chicken soup
15-1/2 oz. can black beans, drained and rinsed
14-oz. can sweet corn & diced peppers, drained
10-oz. can diced tomatoes with green chiles
12-oz. can chicken, drained
8-oz. pkg. pasteurized processed cheese spread, diced

Combine all ingredients except cheese in a stockpot over medium-low heat. Cook, stirring occasionally, for 15 to 20 minutes, until heated through. Add cheese; stir until melted.

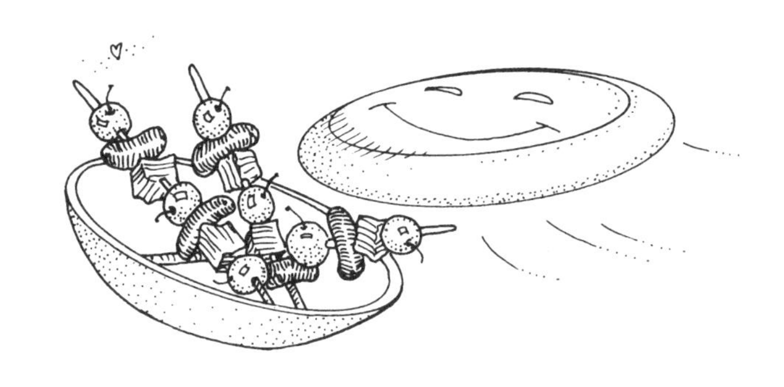

Great for a kids' party...serve finger foods on a plastic flying disc for each child. What fun!

## Incredible Mini Burger Bites

*Makes 24 sandwiches*

2 lbs. lean ground beef
1-1/2 oz. pkg. onion soup mix
2 eggs, beaten
1/2 c. dry bread crumbs
3 T. water
1/2 t. garlic salt
1 t. pepper
24 dinner rolls, split
6 slices American cheese, quartered
Garnish: catsup, mustard, shredded lettuce, thinly sliced onion, dill pickles

Mix first 7 ingredients in a bowl; refrigerate for an hour. Spread beef mixture onto a greased large rimmed baking sheet. Cover with plastic wrap and flatten with a rolling pin. Discard plastic wrap; bake at 400 degrees for 12 minutes. Slice into 24 squares with a pizza cutter. Top each roll with a burger square, a cheese slice and desired garnishes.

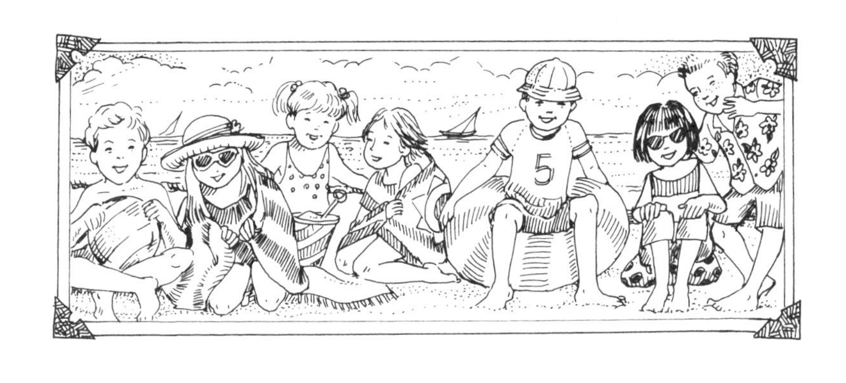


To a young heart, everything is fun.

—Charles Dickens

## Most Bestest Chicken Soup

*Serves 4*

2 chicken breasts
6 c. water
1/2 c. celery, finely chopped
1/2 c. onion, finely chopped
1/2 c. carrots, sliced
4 c. chicken broth
1 c. fine noodles or egg pastina, uncooked
1/8 t. poultry seasoning
salt & pepper to taste

Place chicken breasts and water in a soup pot; cover and bring to a boil. Skim foam from top and sides of pan. Simmer about 45 minutes. Remove chicken and let cool. Skim fat from broth. Add celery, onion, carrots and chicken broth. Simmer 15 minutes. Add noodles or pastina. Meanwhile, remove chicken from bones and chop. Return chicken and seasonings to pot; simmer until noodles are tender and chicken is heated through, about 15 minutes.

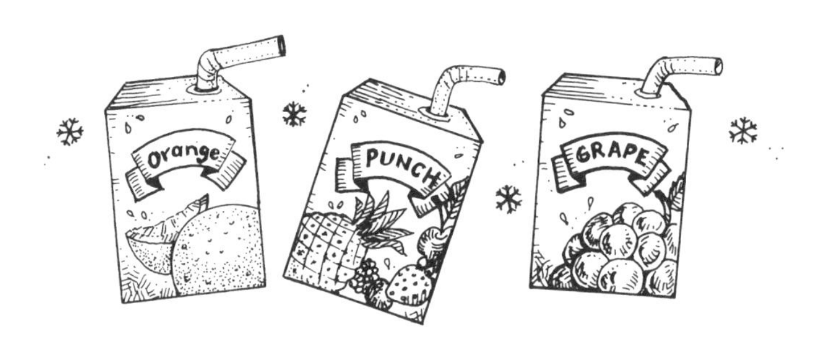


Packing a picnic? Freeze some juice boxes...by the time you're ready to eat, they'll be nice and cool, and they'll help keep the rest of your lunch chilled too!

# Ranch Club Wraps

*Makes 6*

6 leaves green leaf lettuce
6 sandwich wraps
12-oz. pkg. bacon, crisply cooked
1 lb. boneless, skinless chicken
breasts, cooked and shredded
2 tomatoes, diced
ranch salad dressing to taste

Place one leaf lettuce on each sandwich wrap. Top with 2 to 3 slices bacon. Spoon chicken and tomatoes evenly over bacon. Drizzle with salad dressing and roll up.

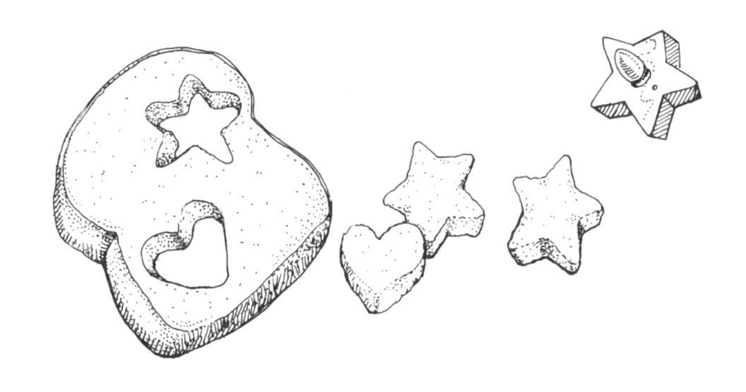

Cute croutons! Butter bread slices and cut into shapes using mini cookie cutters. Bake at 200 degrees until crunchy and golden.

## Cheesy Italiano Soup

*Serves 4*

1-1/4 c. mushrooms, sliced
1/2 c. onion, finely chopped
1 T. oil
2 c. water
15-oz. can pizza sauce
1 c. pepperoni, chopped
1 c. tomatoes, chopped
1/2 c. Italian sausage, cooked
1/4 t. Italian seasoning
1/4 c. grated Parmesan cheese
Garnish: shredded mozzarella cheese

Sauté mushrooms and onion in oil for 2 to 3 minutes, until tender. Add water, pizza sauce, pepperoni, tomatoes, sausage and Italian seasoning. Bring to boil over medium heat; reduce heat and simmer, covered, for 20 minutes. Stir in Parmesan cheese; garnish individual servings with mozzarella.

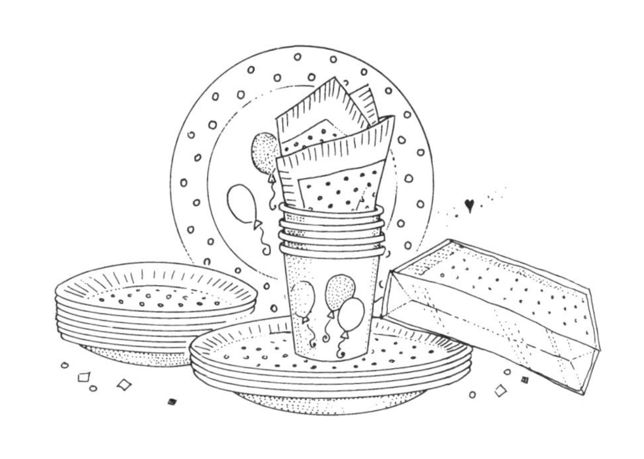

Keep some festive paper plates and napkins tucked away...they'll set a lighthearted mood on busy evenings, plus easy clean-up afterward!

## Corn Dog Muffins

*Makes 6 servings*

8-1/2 oz. pkg. corn muffin mix
1/3 c. water
1 egg, beaten
1/4 c. shredded Cheddar cheese
4 to 6 hot dogs, cut into bite-size pieces
Garnish: catsup, mustard

In a bowl, stir together muffin mix, water and egg. Add cheese and hot dogs; blend together. Fill paper-lined muffin cups 2/3 full. Bake at 400 degrees for 15 to 20 minutes, until golden. Serve with catsup and mustard.

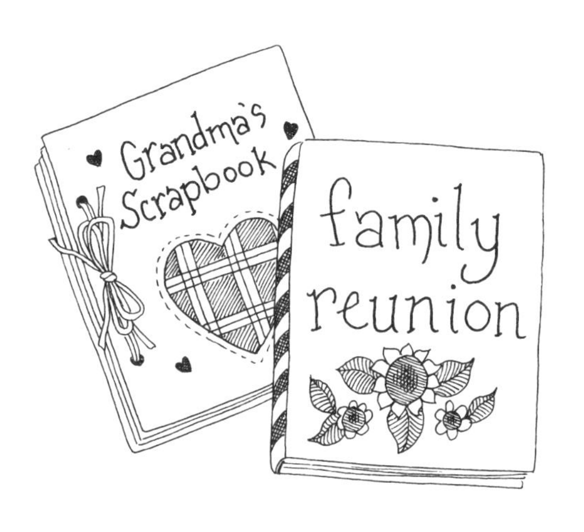


Take time to share family stories and traditions with your kids over the dinner table. A cherished family recipe can be a super conversation starter.

## *Mom's Minestrone*

*Makes 10 to 12 servings*

6 slices bacon
1 onion, chopped
1 c. celery, chopped
2 cloves garlic, minced
2 t. fresh basil, chopped
1/2 t. salt
2 10-3/4 oz. cans bean and bacon soup
2 14-1/2 oz. cans beef broth
2 lbs. canned tomatoes
2 c. zucchini, peeled and chopped
2 c. cabbage, chopped
1 c. macaroni, uncooked
3-3/4 c. water

In a large stockpot, brown bacon, onion, celery and garlic; drain. Add remaining ingredients. Stir well; bring to a boil. Cook, uncovered, for 15 to 20 minutes, until macaroni is tender.

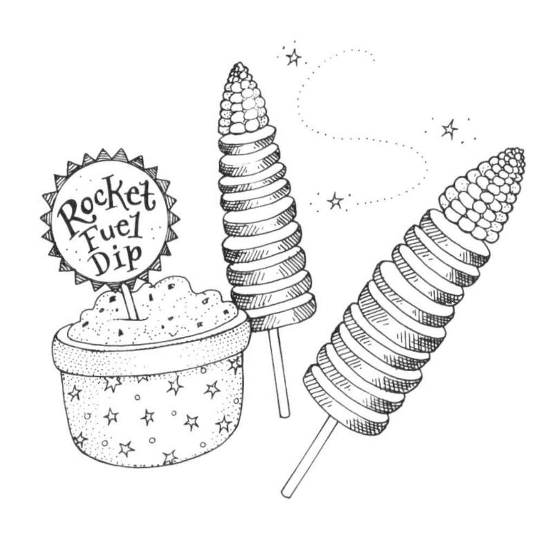


Liven up lunch with Veggie Rockets! Thin slices of carrots, radishes and cucumbers threaded on a skewer make the rocket body; top it off with a baby corncob on the end. Serve with "rocket fuel" dip for a real blast!

## Hamwiches

*Makes 10 servings*

1 loaf frozen bread dough, thawed
2-1/2 c. cooked ham, finely chopped
1 c. shredded Swiss cheese
1 egg yolk
1 T. water

Allow dough to rise according to package directions. Punch down, divide into 10 pieces. Roll each into 5-inch circle. Put 1/4 cup of ham and 2 tablesppons cheese on each circle. Press filling into dough a bit. Beat egg yolk and water together; brush on edges of dough. Fold circles in half; pinch to seal. Brush tops with yolk mixture. Bake at 375 degrees for 15 to 20 minutes on a greased baking sheet, until golden.

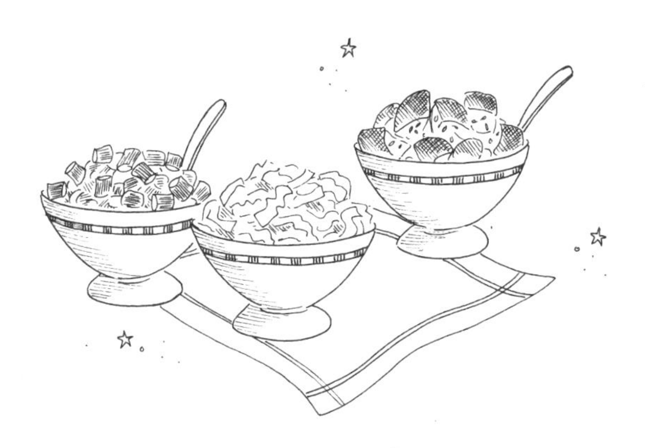

A fun new spin on a "make your own" bar...let kids assemble their own personal lasagna! Use small aluminum loaf pans and set out an assortment of cooked noodles, cooked and crumbled Italian sausage, steamed veggies, spaghetti sauce, ricotta cheese and shredded mozzarella cheese. Place pans on a baking sheet and bake at 300 degrees for 20 minutes.

## One-Pot Chicken & Noodles

*Serves 6*

26-oz. can cream of chicken soup
10-3/4 oz. can cream of mushroom soup
3 14-1/2 oz. cans chicken broth
2 c. cooked chicken breast, diced
2 t. onion powder
1 t. seasoning salt
1/2 t. garlic powder
2 9-oz. pkgs. frozen wide egg noodles, uncooked

Combine soups, broth and chicken in a large pot; bring to a boil over medium-high heat. Add remaining ingredients; reduce heat to low and simmer for 20 to 30 minutes, until noodles are tender.

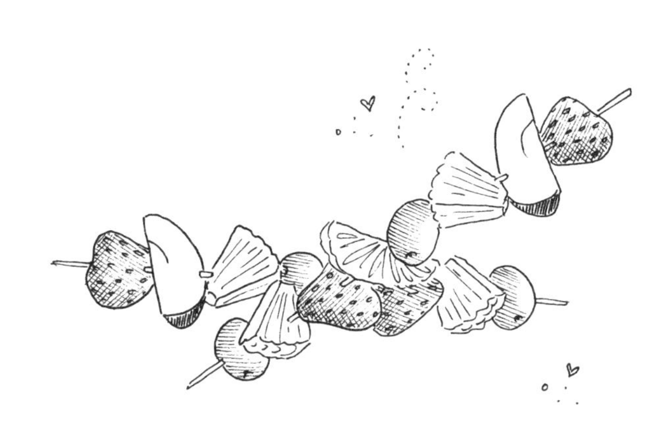

A fresh side dish...fruit kabobs! Just slide pineapple chunks, apple slices, grapes, orange wedges and strawberries onto a wooden skewer.

## Pizza Mac & Cheese

*Makes 8 servings*

7-1/4 oz. pkg. macaroni & cheese
2 eggs, beaten
16-oz. jar pizza sauce
4-oz. pkg. sliced pepperoni
1 c. shredded mozzarella cheese

Prepare macaroni and cheese according to package directions; remove from heat. Add eggs; mix well. Pour into a greased 13"x9" baking pan; bake at 375 degrees for 10 minutes. Spread with pizza sauce; layer pepperoni and mozzarella cheese on top. Return to oven until cheese melts, about 10 minutes.

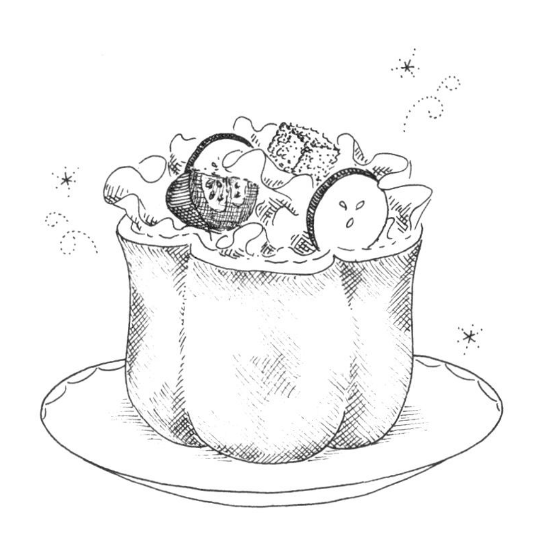

An unexpected side dish...serve up individual servings of crispy salads in hollowed-out red or green peppers.

# *Magic Meatloaf*

*Serves 4 to 6*

2 lbs. ground beef
1 egg, beaten
1/2 c. green pepper, chopped
1/2 c. onion, chopped
1 c. milk
1 c. saltine cracker crumbs
.87-oz. pkg. brown gravy mix
1-1/2 t. salt
6 to 8 new redskin potatoes

Combine all ingredients except potatoes in a large bowl. Mix well and form into a loaf; place in a lightly greased slow cooker. Arrange potatoes around meatloaf. Cover and cook on low setting for 8 to 10 hours, or on high setting for 3 to 5 hours.

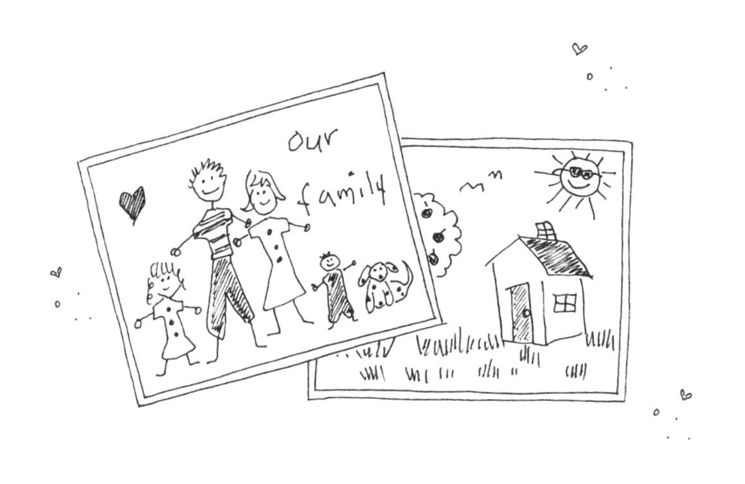


Slip artwork between two pieces of clear self-adhesive plastic for placemats that are both practical and playful.

## Tom Turkey & Stuffing

*Makes 4 to 6 servings*

2 c. cooked turkey, cubed
4 c. assorted frozen vegetables, thawed
10-3/4 oz. can cream of celery soup
10-3/4 oz. can cream of potato soup
1 c. milk
1/4 t. dried thyme
1/8 t. pepper
4 c. sage-flavored stuffing mix, prepared

Arrange turkey in a shallow, ungreased 3-quart casserole dish; top with vegetables. Stir together soups, milk, thyme and pepper in a bowl; spread over turkey and vegetables. Top with stuffing. Bake at 400 degrees for 25 minutes, or until hot.

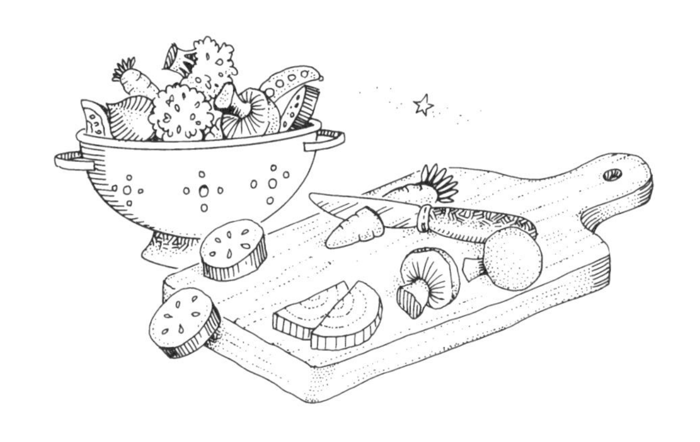

To give a nutritious boost to recipes, add tiny, minced veggies to your family's favorite dishes... they'll blend right in!

## Sloppy Joe Special

*Makes 6 to 12 servings*

8-1/2 oz. pkg. cornbread mix
1/3 c. milk
1 egg, beaten
1 lb. ground beef
6-oz. can tomato paste
1-1/2 oz. pkg. Sloppy Joe seasoning mix
1-1/4 c. water
8-oz. pkg. shredded Cheddar cheese

Prepare cornbread mix with milk and egg according to package directions. Grease the bottom of a 13"x9" baking pan; pour batter into pan. Bake at 350 degrees for 8 minutes, or until golden. Meanwhile, brown beef in a skillet over medium heat; drain. Stir in tomato paste, seasoning mix and water; bring to a boil. Reduce heat and let simmer for 5 minutes. Spoon beef mixture over warm cornbread; sprinkle with cheese. Place under broiler just long enough to melt cheese. Cut into squares to serve.

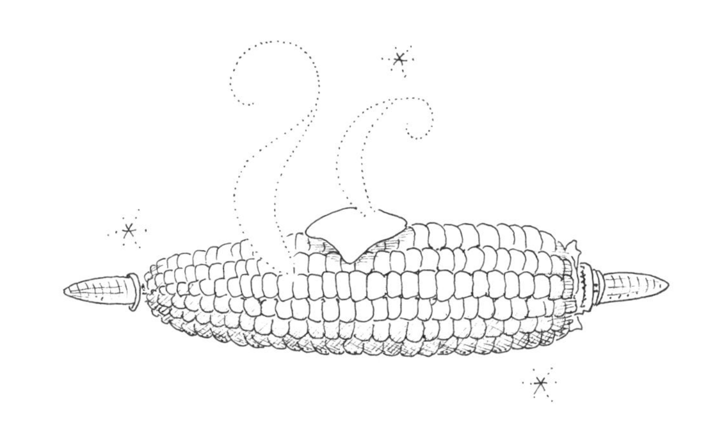

Kids love corn on the cob...and it can be ready in just four minutes! Simply place husked ears of corn under a broiler, turning as needed, until golden on all sides.

## Cheeseburger & Fries Casserole

*Makes 6 to 8 servings*

2 lbs. ground beef, browned and drained
10-3/4 oz. can golden mushroom soup
10-3/4 oz. can Cheddar cheese soup
20-oz. pkg. frozen crinkle-cut French fries

Combine beef and soups; spread in a greased 13"x9" baking pan. Arrange French fries on top. Bake, uncovered, at 350 degrees for 50 to 55 minutes, until fries are golden.

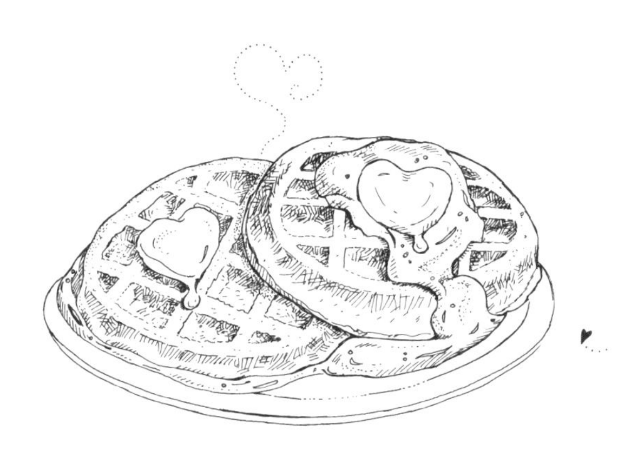

A fun new way to serve cornbread...mix up the batter, thin it slightly with a little extra milk, then bake until crisp in a waffle iron.

## *Mexican Lasagna*

*Makes 12 servings*

10 flour tortillas, quartered
1 lb. ground beef, browned
1 c. salsa
15-oz. can tomato sauce
1-1/4 oz. pkg. taco seasoning
16-oz. container cottage cheese
1 T. dried oregano
2 eggs, beaten
1-1/2 c. mozzarella cheese

Layer 1/2 of tortilla quarters in a lightly greased 13"x9" baking dish; set aside. Combine beef, salsa, tomato sauce and taco seasoning; layer half over tortillas. In a separate bowl, combine cottage cheese, oregano and eggs; layer over beef mixture. Spread remaining beef mixture on top; layer remaining tortilla quarters over beef mixture. Sprinkle with mozzarella cheese; bake at 375 degrees for 30 minutes, or until hot and bubbly.

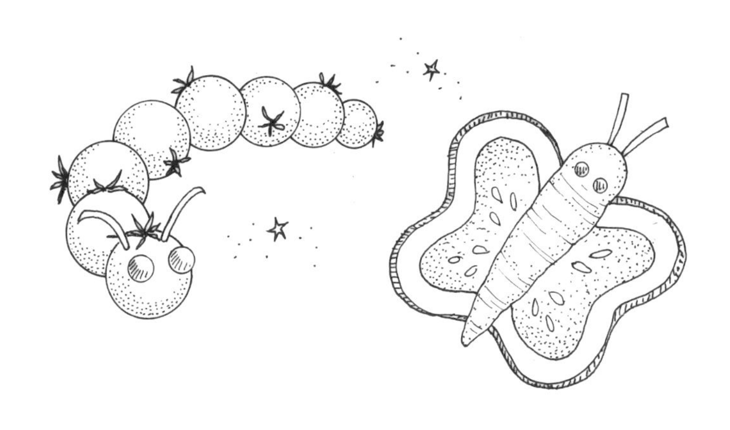

Eat your veggies! With an assortment of bite-sized vegetables and using flavored cream cheese as "glue," kids can create their very own "critter snack attack."

## Crispy Chicken Bites

*Serves 4*

1-1/2 c. corn flake cereal, crushed
1 t. paprika
1/2 t. Italian seasoning
1/4 t. garlic powder
1/4 t. onion powder
salt and pepper to taste
1/2 c. milk
2 boneless, skinless chicken breasts, cut into 2-inch pieces
1/4 c. butter, melted
Garnish: favorite dipping sauce

Combine cereal and seasonings in a shallow bowl; set aside. Pour milk into a separate bowl. Dip chicken pieces into milk, then into cereal mixture and coat thoroughly. Place in single layer on a baking sheet sprayed with non-stick vegetable spray. Drizzle butter over chicken and sprinkle with additional salt, if desired. Bake at 350 degrees for 15 to 20 minutes, until no longer pink in the middle. Serve with your favorite sauce.

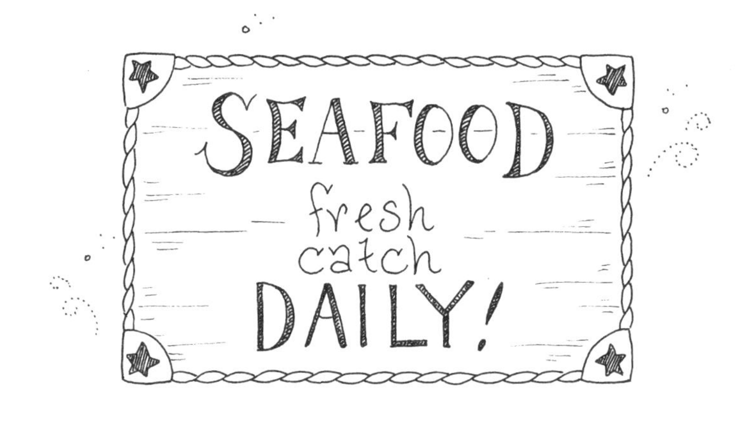


A handy tip to make frozen fish taste fresh and mild... just place the frozen fillets in a shallow dish, cover with milk and thaw in the refrigerator overnight.

## Super-Fast Tilapia Parmesan

*Makes 8 servings*

1/2 c. grated Parmesan cheese
1/4 c. butter, softened
3 T. mayonnaise
2 T. lemon juice
1/4 t. dried basil
1/4 t. pepper
1/8 t. onion powder
1/8 t. celery salt
2 lbs. tilapia fillets

In a small bowl, blend together all ingredients except fish fillets; set aside. Arrange fillets in a single layer on a lightly greased broiler pan. Broil on top rack of oven for 2 to 3 minutes. Turn and broil other side for 2 to 3 minutes. Remove from oven; top fish with Parmesan mixture. Broil for 2 additional minutes, or until topping is golden and fish flakes easily with a fork.

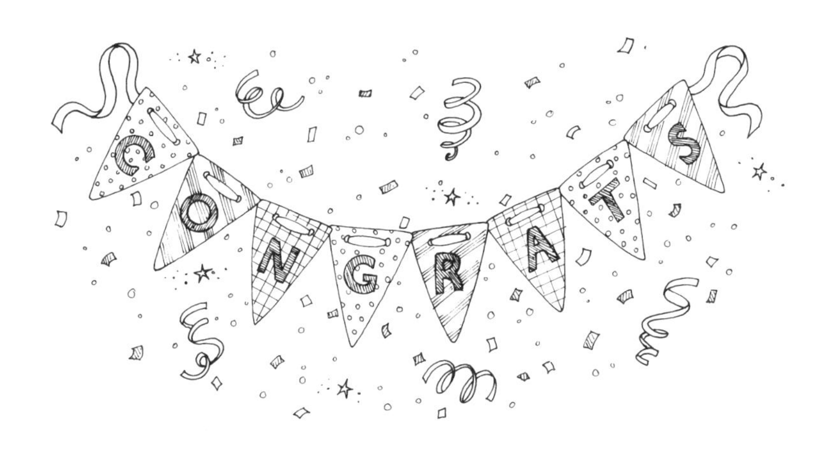


Find a reason to celebrate! Kids will love it when you recognize their achievements...an A in math, the game-winning goal or a new Scout badge...in a big way.

## Lasagna Toss

*Serves 6*

1/2 lb. ground beef
1/2 lb. ground Italian pork sausage
1/2 c. onion, chopped
1/2 t. salt
1/8 t. garlic powder
1-3/4 c. spaghetti sauce
8-oz. pkg. mafalda pasta or broken lasagna noodles, cooked
1 c. cottage cheese
2 c. shredded mozzarella cheese

In a large skillet over medium heat, brown ground beef, sausage, onion, salt and garlic powder; drain. Stir in sauce; simmer until heated through. Stir in pasta and cottage cheese. Spoon into a lightly greased 2-quart casserole dish; top with mozzarella cheese. Bake, uncovered, at 350 degrees for 20 to 25 minutes.

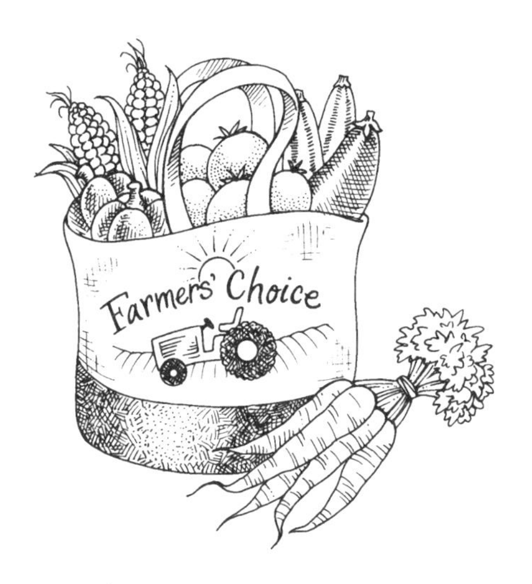


Include kids in the weekly meal planning, preparation and clean-up. When kids are involved, they're more likely to eat what's served!

## Cheesy Ham & Vegetable Bake

*Serves 6*

1-1/2 c. rotini pasta, uncooked
16-oz. pkg. frozen broccoli, carrot and cauliflower blend
1/2 c. sour cream
1/2 c. milk
1-1/2 c. shredded Cheddar cheese, divided
1-1/2 c. cooked ham, chopped
1/4 c. onion, chopped
1 clove garlic, minced
1/2 c. croutons, crushed

Cook pasta according to package directions; add frozen vegetables to cooking water just to thaw. Drain; place mixture in a 2-quart casserole dish that has been sprayed with non-stick vegetable spray. Mix sour cream, milk, one cup cheese, ham, onion and garlic; stir into pasta mixture. Bake, uncovered, at 350 degrees for 30 minutes. Sprinkle with croutons and remaining cheese during last 5 minutes of baking.

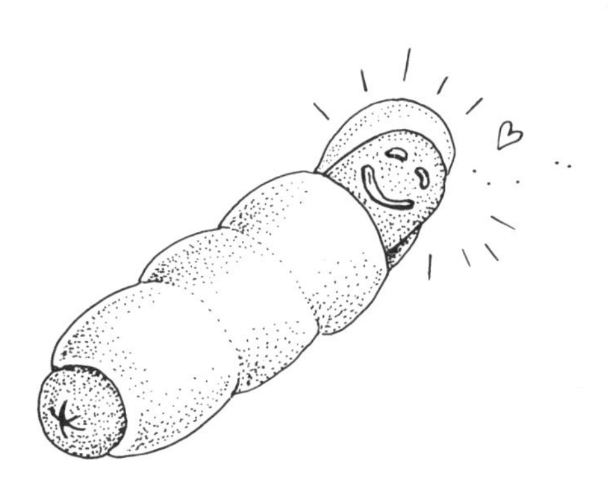

How spooky...mummy dogs! Simply wrap a strip of breadstick dough around individual hot dogs. Arrange them on an ungreased baking sheet and bake at 375 degrees for 12 to 15 minutes. Add eyes with dots of catsup or mustard.

## Chinese Fried Rice

*Makes 4 to 6 servings*

3 T. oil
1 c. cooked chicken, pork or shrimp, chopped
2 eggs, beaten
3/4 t. salt
1/2 t. pepper
3 c. cooked rice, chilled
2 T. soy sauce
Garnish: 2 green onions, snipped

Heat oil in a deep skillet over medium heat. Add meat and cook for one minute. Add eggs, salt and pepper; cook, stirring constantly, until eggs are set. Add rice and soy sauce; cook, stirring constantly, for about 5 minutes, until rice is heated through. Garnish with green onions.

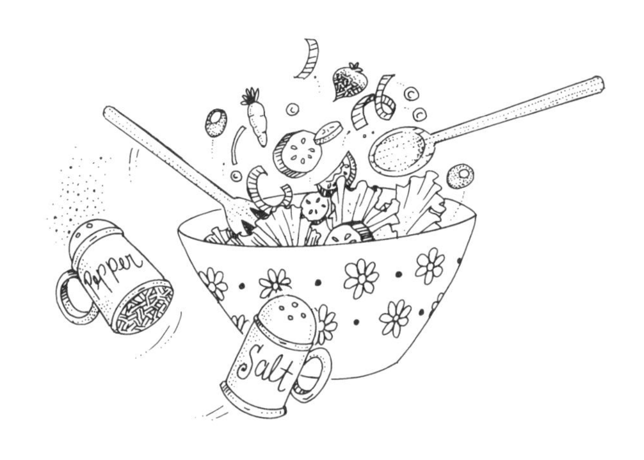


Let the rest of the family help! Younger children can tear lettuce for salad...older kids can measure and chop ingredients or stir a skillet.

## Wacky Beef Roast

*Serves 6*

2 to 3-lb. beef chuck roast
1-oz. pkg. ranch dressing mix
.7-oz. pkg. Italian dressing mix
.87-oz. pkg. brown gravy mix
1/2 to 1 c. warm water

Place roast in a slow cooker. Combine dry dressing and gravy mixes; sprinkle over roast. Pour in warm water. Cover and cook on low setting for 6 to 8 hours.

Make the family tree more interesting! Hang color copies of photos on a white-washed branch that's been tucked in a sap bucket. Show the kids Aunt Lucille or Uncle Bob...it will make sharing family stories much more fun.

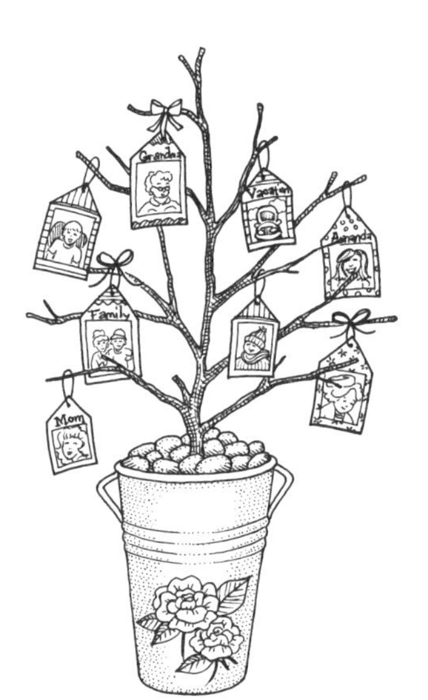

## *Family Favorite Corn Soufflé*

*Serves 12 to 14*

15-oz. can corn, drained
8-1/2 oz. pkg. cornbread mix
14-3/4 oz. can creamed corn
1 c. sour cream
1/4 c. butter, melted
8-oz. pkg. shredded Cheddar cheese

Combine all ingredients except cheese. Pour into a lightly greased 13"x9" glass baking pan. Cover with aluminum foil. Bake at 350 degrees for 30 minutes. Uncover and add cheese. Return to oven and continue baking until cheese is bubbly and golden, about 15 minutes.

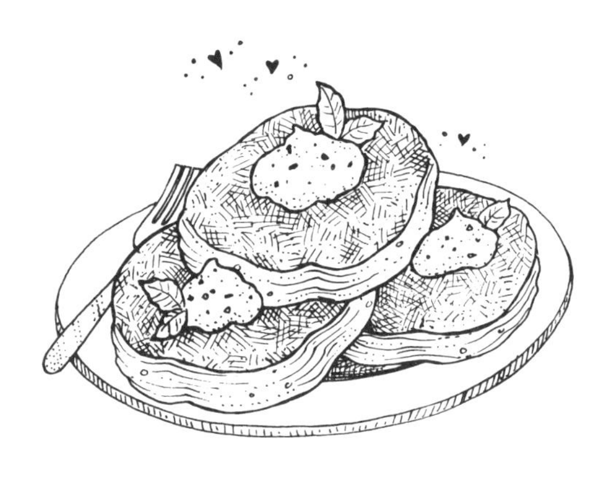

Make crispy potato pancakes with extra mashed potatoes. Stir an egg yolk and some minced onion into 2 cups cold mashed potatoes. Form into patties, dust with a little flour and pan-fry in a little oil until golden.

## Snowy White Mashed Potatoes

*Serves 8 to 10*

5 lbs. potatoes, peeled, cooked and mashed
1 c. sour cream
8-oz. pkg. cream cheese, softened
1/4 c. butter, melted
1/4 t. granulated garlic
1 t. salt
1 t. pepper
1/8 t. dried parsley
3 T. butter, sliced
1/8 t. paprika

In a medium bowl, beat together all ingredients except butter and paprika. Spoon potatoes into a greased 2-quart casserole dish. Dot potatoes with butter. Sprinkle paprika over top. Bake, covered, at 350 degrees for 25 minutes.

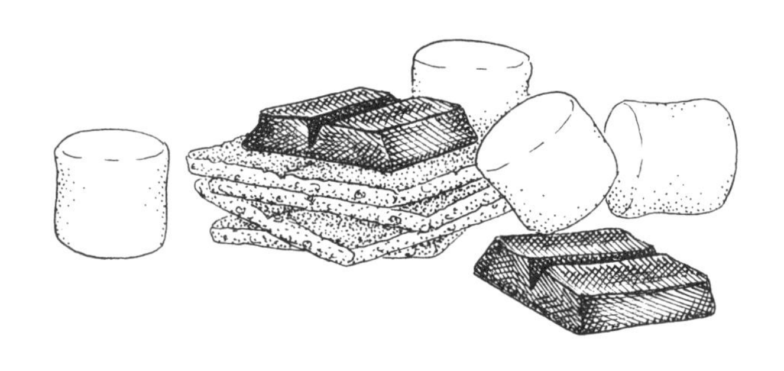

To make easy s'mores, wrap up your ingredients in a square of aluminum foil, sealing the edges well. Toss on the outer edges of your bonfire and let sit 5 minutes or until chocolate and marshmallows have melted. Unwrap and enjoy!

## Campfire Veggies

*Serves 4*

1 onion, thinly sliced
4 potatoes, thinly sliced
1 c. carrot, peeled and thinly sliced
1 c. green beans, trimmed
1 T. butter
1/8 t. dill weed or favorite dried herb
Optional: 1 clove garlic, chopped

In the center of a large sheet of heavy-duty aluminum foil, layer all ingredients in order given. Fold and seal edges of foil around mixture to create a packet. Place packet on a campfire grate or outdoor grill. Cook over medium heat for about 25 to 30 minutes.

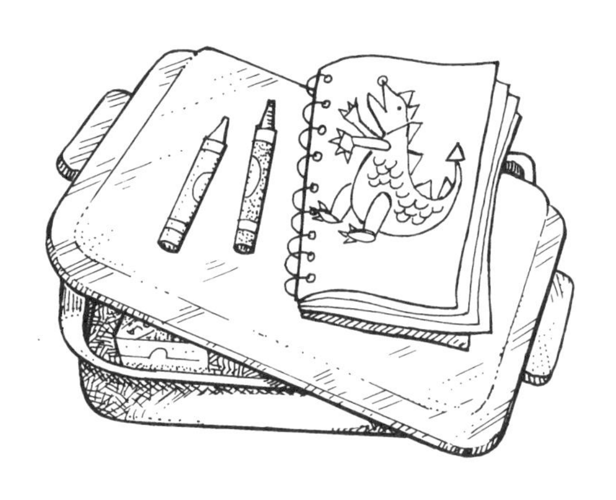

A rectangular cake pan with its own lid makes a great lap tray for kids in the car...fill it with crayons, paper and small treats.

## Kids' Favorite Fruit Salad

*Serves 6 to 8*

14-1/2 oz. can peach pie filling
1 c. pineapple tidbits
1 c. seedless red grapes
2 bananas, sliced
11-oz. can mandarin oranges, drained
1 c. mini marshmallows

Mix all ingredients together in a large bowl; refrigerate until chilled.

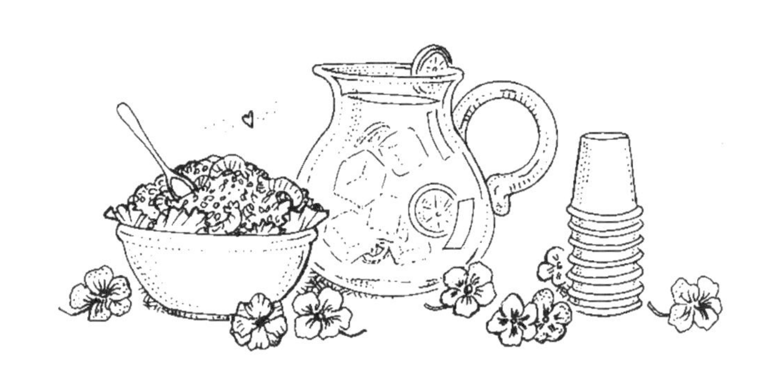

Example is contagious behavior.

—C. Reade

## *Sunny Lemonade Salad*

*Makes 6 to 8 servings*

15-1/4 oz. can crushed pineapple, drained
14-oz. can sweetened condensed milk
6-oz. can frozen lemonade concentrate, thawed
8-oz. container frozen whipped topping, thawed
2 c. mini marshmallows

Combine pineapple, milk and lemonade; fold in whipped topping and marshmallows. Cover and chill until time to serve.

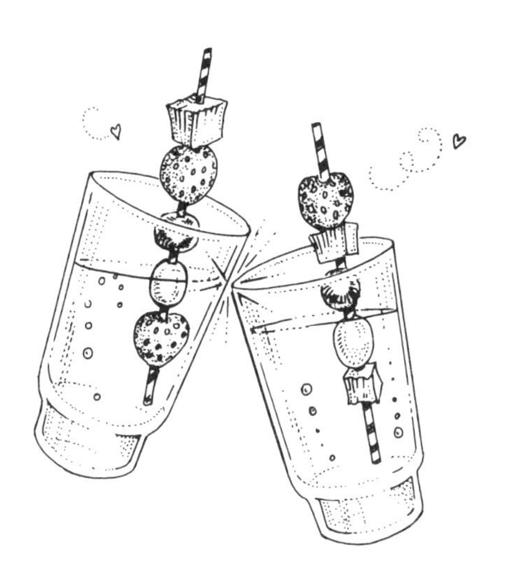

Turn fruit juice into a special-occasion beverage...add a splash of ginger ale and a skewer of fruit cubes lined up on a plastic straw.

## Cheddar Cheesy Bread

*Makes one loaf*

2 c. all-purpose flour
1 T. sugar
1 T. baking powder
1/2 t. salt
1/4 c. butter
3/4 c. milk
1 egg, beaten
1 c. sharp Cheddar cheese, shredded

Coat a 8"x4" loaf pan with non-stick vegetable spray; set aside. Stir together flour, sugar, baking powder and salt. Cut in butter until mixture resembles coarse crumbs. Stir milk and egg into flour mixture; add Cheddar cheese. Stir well and pour batter into prepared pan. Bake at 350 degrees for 35 minutes, or until golden.

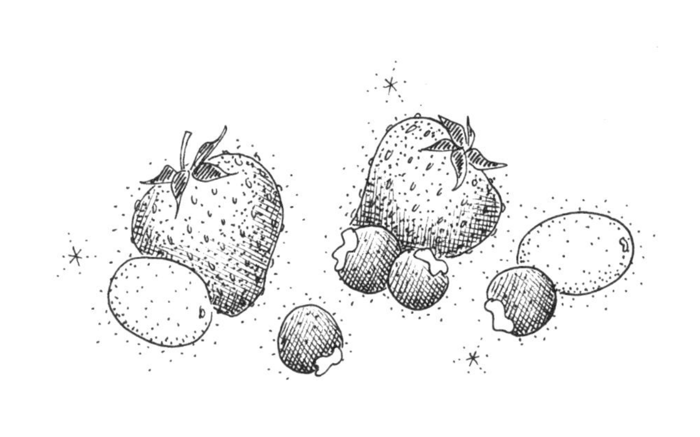

An edible, glittery garnish...roll grapes, strawberries
and blueberries in extra-fine sugar.
Kids will eat 'em up!

## ABC Salad

*Makes 6 to 8 servings*

1/2 c. canola oil
1/4 c. lemon juice, divided
1 t. sugar
1/4 t. salt
1 c. sweetened dried cranberries
3 red apples, cored and cut into 1/2-inch cubes
2 c. broccoli flowerets
1/2 c. chopped walnuts

In a bowl, whisk together oil, 2 tablespoons lemon juice, sugar and salt. Add cranberries; let stand for 10 minutes. In a large bowl, toss apples with remaining lemon juice. Add broccoli, walnuts and cranberry mixture; toss to coat. Cover and refrigerate for 2 hours, or until chilled. Toss before serving.

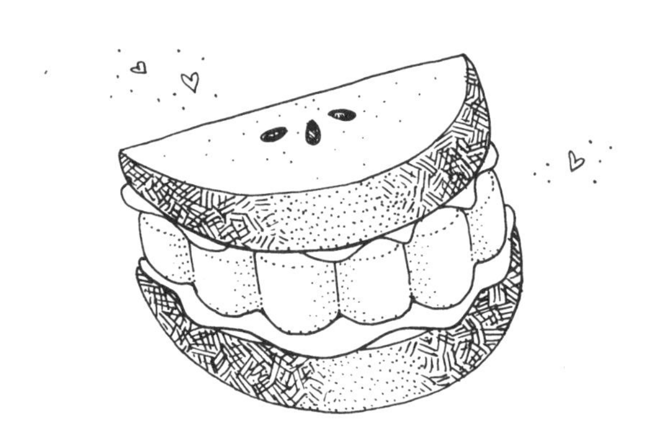

Make "apple smiles" with your little ones! Cut washed apples into eight wedges. Spread peanut butter on one side of each slice. Place mini marshmallows on the peanut butter for teeth. Place another peanut-buttered apple slice on top so the peel sides match and the marshmallows are sandwiched between apples.

## Fairy Bread

*Makes one loaf*

1-lb. loaf frozen bread dough
1/4 c. flour
red, blue & purple food coloring

Thaw dough and allow to rise according to package instructions. Divide dough into 3 equal parts. Add 5 drops of each color of food coloring to the dough: one part red, one blue, on purple. Knead well and then let dough rest on a floured baking sheet. Divide each ball of dough into 2 pieces. Flatten it out until it's about 8 inches long, then stack the pieces on top of each other, alternating the colors. Fold ends of dough into the middle. Place dough in an 8"x4" loaf pan that's been sprayed with non-stick vegetable spray. Let dough rest again for about an hour, until it rises an inch or so above the pan. Bake at 350 degrees for 25 to 30 minutes. Remove from pan immediately and allow to cool before slicing.

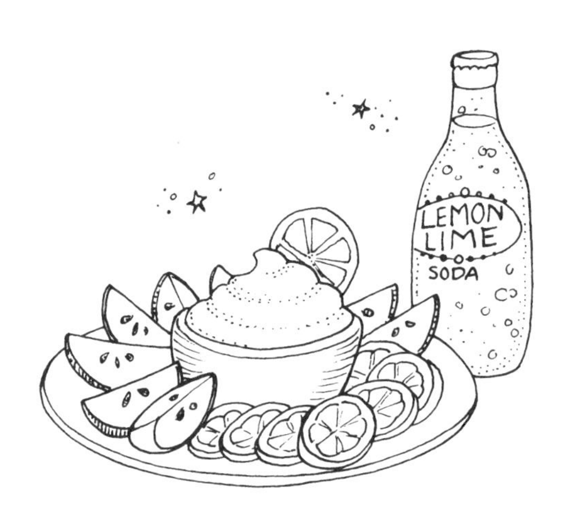


To keep just-cut fruit slices looking fresh, dip them into lemon-lime soda before serving.

## Apple Wheels

*Makes 4 servings*

1/4 c. creamy peanut butter
2 t. honey
1/2 c. semi-sweet mini chocolate chips
1 T. raisins
4 red or yellow apples, cored

Combine peanut butter and honey in a bowl; fold in chocolate chips and raisins. Fill centers of apples with mixture; refrigerate for one hour. Slice apples into 1/4-inch rings to serve.

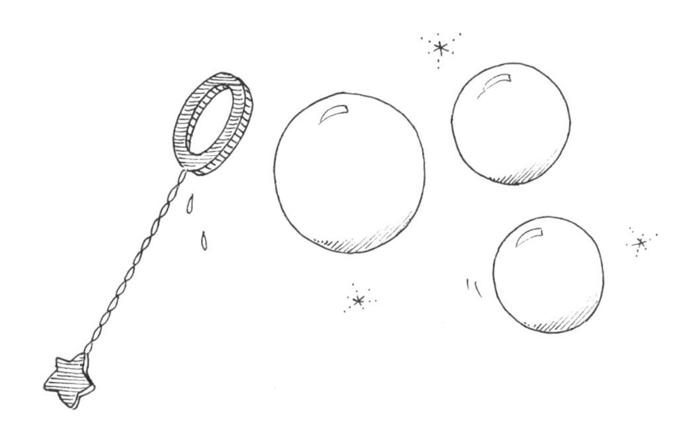

Oodles of bubbles! For an easy homemade bubble solution, just mix 10 cups of water with 4 cups dishwashing liquid and one cup of corn syrup.

## Make-Believe Champagne

*Makes 20 servings*

1-ltr. bottle carbonated water, chilled
1-ltr. bottle ginger ale, chilled
24-oz. bottle unsweetened white grape juice, chilled
ice cubes

In a large pitcher, combine carbonated water, ginger ale and white grape juice. Pour over ice cubes in chilled stemmed glasses.

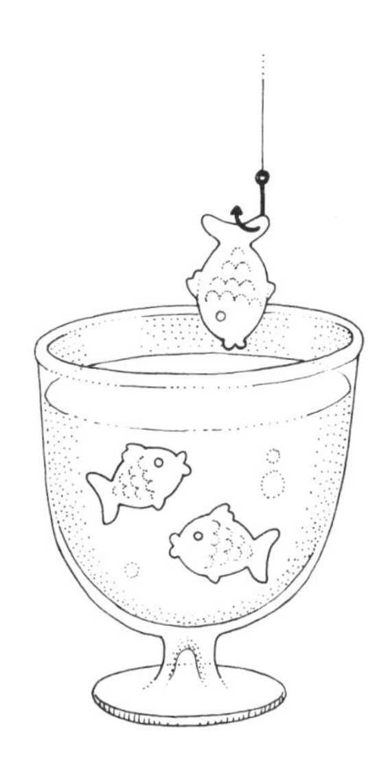

Something fishy is going on in dessert-land! Fill clear cups with blue gelatin and let the kids drop in gummy fish.

## Tropical Whip Fruit Dip

*Serves 4 to 6*

1 c. cream cheese, softened
1 c. pineapple yogurt
1 c. frozen whipped topping, thawed
1/4 c. coconut
1/4 c. chopped pecans
fruit, pretzels or cookies for dipping

Beat cream cheese until fluffy with an electric mixer set on low. Add yogurt a little at a time. Fold in whipped topping, coconut and pecans; stir well. Chill at least 15 minutes before serving.

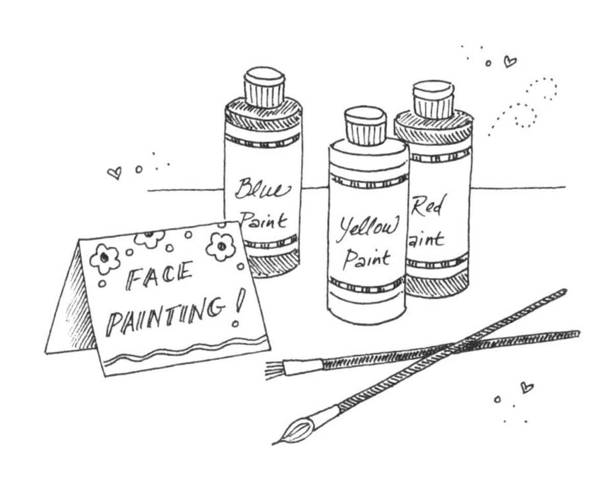


Mix up your own face paints! All you need is 1 teaspoon cornstarch, 1/2 teaspoon cold cream, 1/2 teaspoon cold water and the desired amount of food coloring. Combine all ingredients. Later, remove face paint with cold cream.

## Mac & Cheese Nuggets

*Makes 4 dozen*

1/4 c. grated Parmesan cheese, divided
1-1/2 T. butter
2 T. all-purpose flour
3/4 c. milk
1-1/4 c. shredded Cheddar cheese
1/4 lb. American cheese slices, chopped
1 egg yolk, beaten
1/4 t. paprika
8-oz. pkg. elbow macaroni, cooked

Lightly grease mini muffin cups. Sprinkle with 2 tablespoons Parmesan cheese, tapping out excess. Melt butter in a large saucepan over medium heat. Stir in flour; cook for 2 minutes. Whisk in milk until boiling, about 5 minutes. Add Cheddar and American cheeses; remove from heat and stir until smooth. Whisk in egg yolk and paprika; fold in macaroni until well coated. Spoon rounded tablespoons of mixture into prepared tins; sprinkle with remaining Parmesan. Bake at 425 degrees for 10 minutes, or until hot and golden. Cool for 5 minutes; carefully transfer to a serving plate.

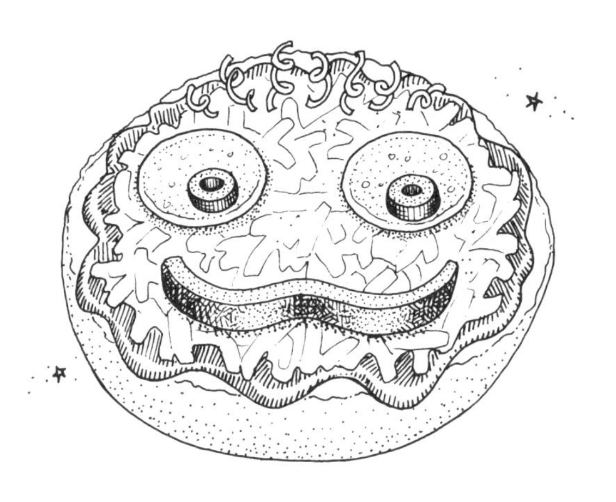

Freaky-face pizza snacks! Lightly toast English muffin halves, spread with pizza sauce, and sprinkle with cheese. Make a face with toppings such as pepperoni and black olive "eyes," carrot curl "hair" and green pepper "smiles."

## Strawberry-Watermelon Slush *Makes 5 to 6 servings*

1 pt. strawberries, hulled and halved
2 c. watermelon, seeded and cubed
1/3 c. sugar
1/3 c. lemon juice
2 c. ice cubes

Combine strawberries, watermelon, sugar and lemon juice in a blender. Blend until smooth. Gradually add ice and continue to blend. Serve immediately.

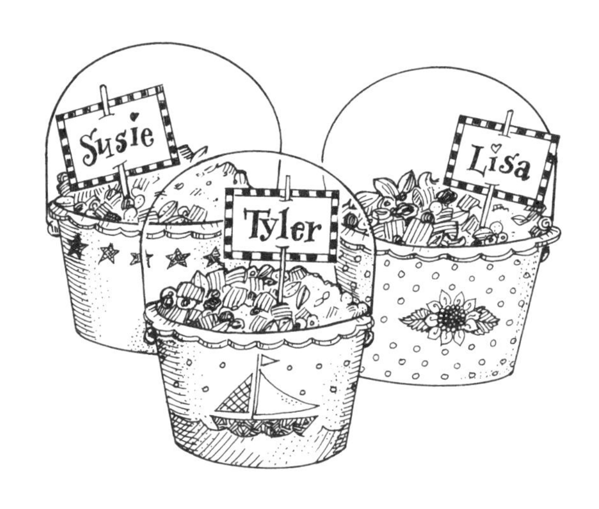


New plastic pails make whimsical picnic servers for party chips and snacks. Afterward, the kids can use them for treasure hunting around the backyard.

## Maple Popcorn Balls

*Makes about one dozen*

24 c. popped popcorn
2 c. golden raisins
2 c. chopped nuts
2/3 c. maple syrup
1-1/2 t. maple extract
2/3 c. apple juice
1/2 c. butter, sliced
3/4 t. salt
2 c. sugar

Combine popcorn, raisins and nuts in a large bowl; set aside. Mix remaining ingredients in a large heavy saucepan. Cook and stir over medium heat until sugar dissolves. If mixture tries to rise above pan, lower heat. Watch closely, as temperature will rise very quickly toward the end. Stop stirring just before mixture reaches hard-crack stage, or 290 to 310 degrees on a candy thermometer. Immediately remove from heat and pour over popcorn mixture; stir to coat. Working quickly with buttered hands, form into tennis ball-sized balls. Cool; wrap in cellophane.

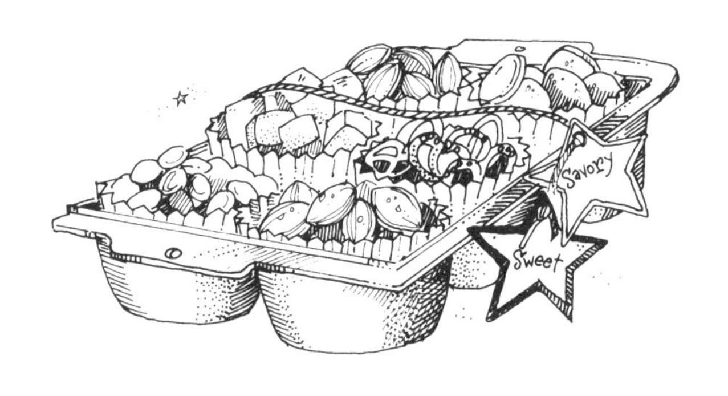


Fill a muffin tray with different veggies, fruits, nuts and dips for a fresh snack.

## PB&J Milkshakes

*Makes one serving*

2 T. creamy peanut butter
3 T. favorite-flavor jelly
1/2 c. milk
1 c. vanilla ice cream

Stir peanut butter and jelly together in a small bowl. Add milk and ice cream to a blender; add peanut butter mixture. Blend until smooth. Serve immediately.

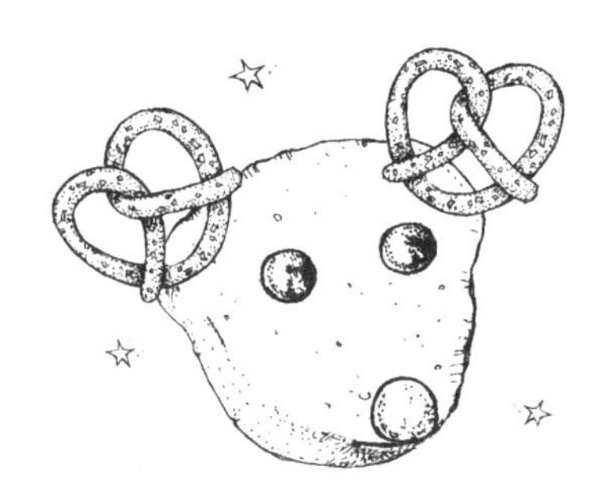

Kids will love these sweet reindeer cookies! Start with your favorite plain drop cookie dough recipe and shape into one-inch balls. Pinch the ball to form a point and gently flatten with your hand. Bake as directed. Remove from oven; immediately press two mini chocolate-covered pretzels into the tops of the cookies for the antlers, two mini brown candy-coated chocolates for the eyes and a regular-sized red candy-coated chocolate for the nose.

## Pizza Roll Snacks

*Makes 16*

8-oz. tube refrigerated crescent rolls
1/3 c. pizza sauce
1/4 c. grated Parmesan cheese
16 slices pepperoni, divided
1/3 c. shredded mozzarella cheese, divided

Unroll rolls but do not separate; press perforations to seal. Spread pizza sauce evenly over rolls, leaving a one-inch border. Sprinkle with Parmesan cheese. Roll up dough jelly-roll fashion, starting with the short side. Using a sharp knife, cut into 15 slices. Place slices cut-side down on a greased baking sheet. Top each slice with one pepperoni slice and one teaspoon mozzarella cheese. Bake at 375 degrees for 9 to 11 minutes, until edges are golden and cheese is melted.

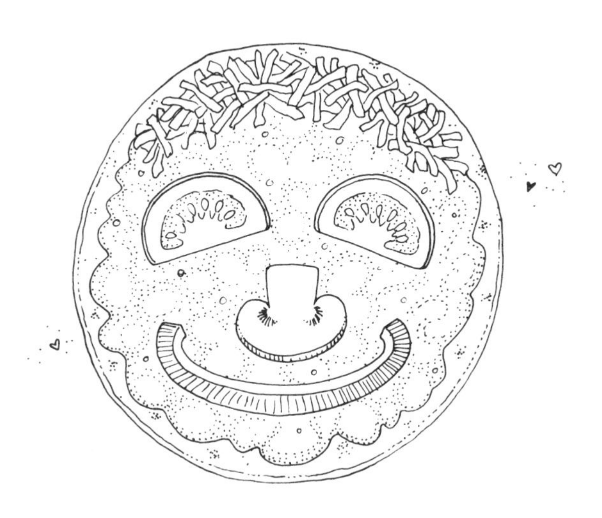

Spread refried beans on an open tortilla, and use shredded lettuce for "hair" and bits of fresh veggies for features on a happy face tortilla treat.

## Fiesta Pinwheels

*Makes 4 to 6 servings*

16-oz. can refried beans
1/4 c. salsa
2 T. taco seasoning
1 c. sour cream
6 to 8 8-inch flour tortillas
1/4 c. sliced black olives
8-oz. pkg. shredded Mexican-blend cheese

Mix together beans, salsa and seasoning; set aside. Spread one tablespoon sour cream on each tortilla; top with 2 tablespoons bean mixture. Sprinkle each with black olives and cheese. Roll tightly and cut into bite-size pieces.

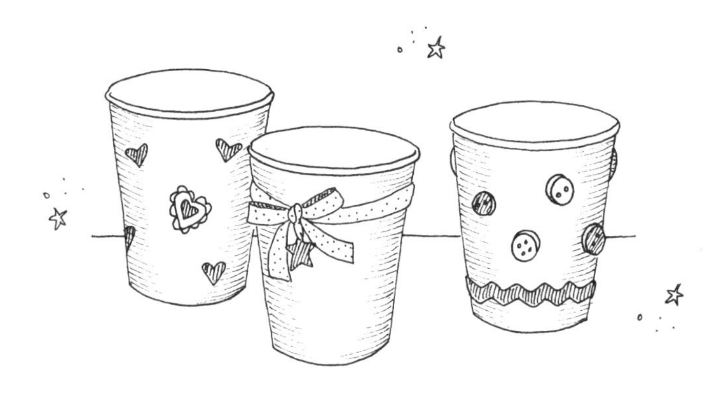

Using paper cups? Embellish them with fun touches kids big and little will love! Faux jewels, stickers, wax seals and ribbon easily turn plain paper cups into something special.

## Oh-So-Easy Apple Cider

*Makes about 40 servings*

3 qts. apple juice
2 qts. cranberry juice cocktail
1/2 c. brown sugar, packed
4 4-inch cinnamon sticks

Mix all ingredients together in a large stockpot. Simmer over low heat until hot; serve warm.

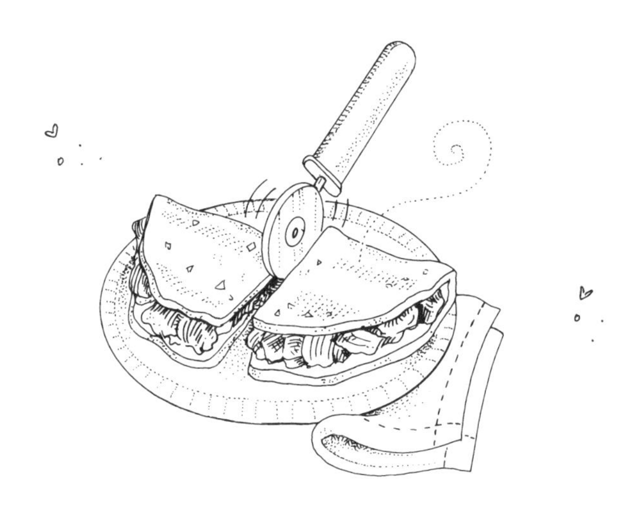

Make your pizza cutter do double duty...it's oh-so handy for slicing cheesy quesadillas into wedges too.

## Cheesy Chicken Quesadillas

*Serves 4*

8 8-inch flour tortillas, divided
1/2 c. ranch salad dressing
1 c. shredded Monterey Jack cheese
1 c. shredded Cheddar cheese
12-1/2 oz. can chicken, drained
1/3 c. bacon bits
Garnish: salsa

Spread 4 tortillas evenly with salad dressing. Layer with cheeses, chicken, bacon and remaining tortillas. Place each quesadilla into a skillet sprayed with non-stick vegetable spray. Grill over medium-high heat for about 2 minutes on each side, or until golden and cheese is melted. Let stand for 2 minutes; cut into wedges. Serve with salsa.

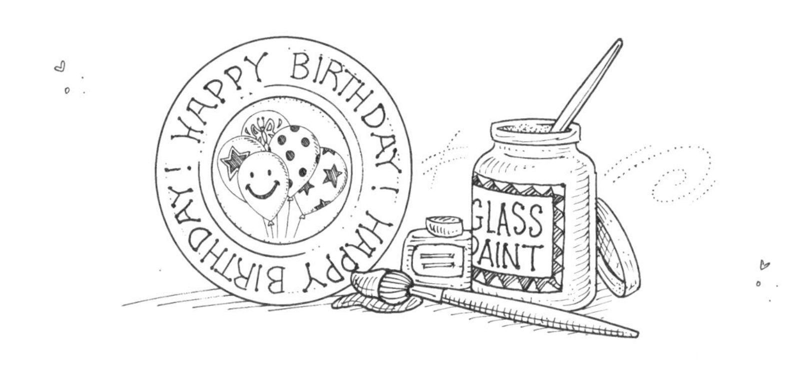


Make a celebration plate for serving up special treats. Check your local craft store for a clear glass plate and for craft paints designed especially for glass. Along the rim of the plate, add a special message like "Happy Birthday" or "Congratulations."

## Monster Cookies

*Makes 3 dozen*

3 eggs, beaten
1-1/2 c. brown sugar, packed
1 c. white sugar
3/4 t. vanilla extract
1 t. light corn syrup
2 t. baking soda
1/2 c. margarine, softened
1-1/2 c. creamy peanut butter
4-1/2 c. quick-cooking oats, uncooked
2/3 c. semi-sweet chocolate chips
2/3 c. candy-coated chocolate pieces

In a large bowl, combine all ingredients in order given. Drop by rounded teaspoonfuls onto ungreased cookie sheets. Flatten slightly. Bake at 350 degrees for 10 minutes. Cool on baking sheet for 3 minutes; transfer to wire racks.

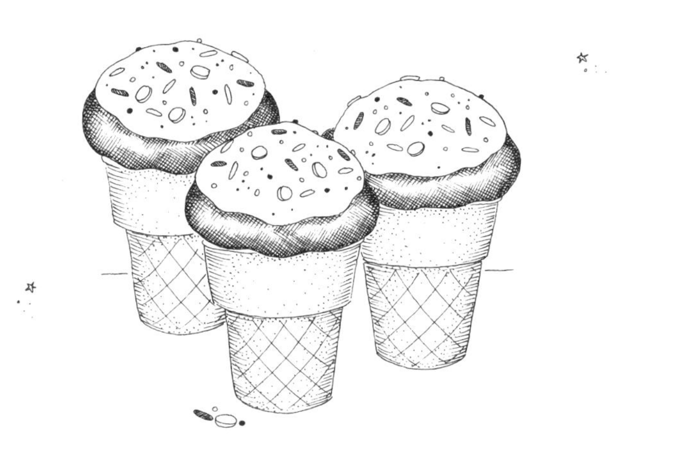

Make cupcake cones! Fill ice cream cones with cake batter to within 1/2 inch of the top; carefully arrange in an ungreased muffin tin. Bake at 375 degrees for 35 minutes; cool completely on wire racks. Frost and decorate as desired.

## *S'mores Pudding Pie*

*Makes 8 servings*

7-oz. jar marshmallow creme
9-inch graham cracker crust
3.9-oz. pkg. instant chocolate pudding mix
1 c. hard-shell chocolate topping
Optional: whipped topping, mini chocolate chips

Spread marshmallow creme gently in crust and set aside. Prepare pudding mix according to package instructions; pour pudding over marshmallow creme. Spread topping over pie. Chill for 1-1/2 hours. If desired, garnish with dollops of whipped topping and a sprinkle of mini chocolate chips.

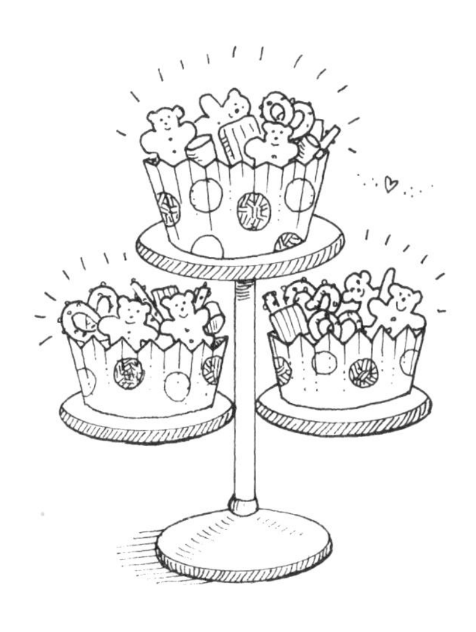

Serve up individual servings of snack mix in colorful cupcake wrappers. Stack them on a tiered cupcake stand for a fun party decoration!

## *Mom's Puppy Chow*

*Makes 10 servings*

16-oz. pkg. bite-size crispy corn cereal squares
1 c. sugar
1 c. corn syrup
1 c. creamy peanut butter
1 c. dry-roasted peanuts

Place cereal in a large bowl; set aside. In a microwave-safe bowl, combine sugar, corn syrup and peanut butter. Microwave on high until melted, about 3 minutes. Add peanuts; mix well and pour over cereal. Toss evenly to coat. Store in an airtight container.

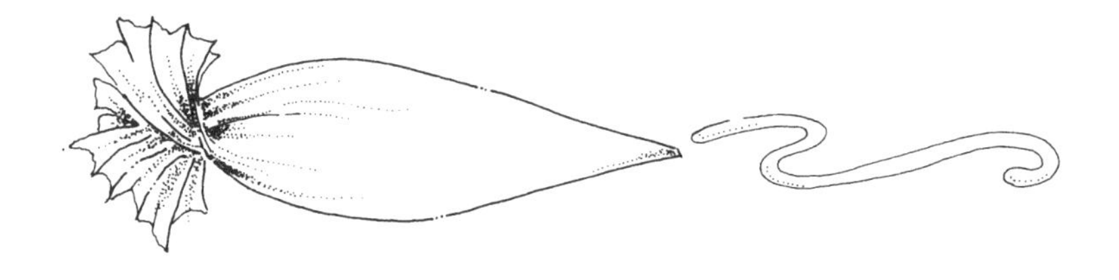

Easy-squeezy! Place frosting ingredients in a plastic zipping bag. Squeeze to mix well, then snip off a small corner and squeeze to drizzle over baked goods.

## Quick Apple Dumplings

*Serves 8*

8-oz. tube refrigerated crescent rolls
2 Granny Smith apples, cored, peeled and quartered
1/8 t. cinnamon
1/2 c. butter
1 c. sugar
1 c. orange juice
1 t. vanilla extract
1/2 c. pecans, very finely chopped
Optional: ice cream

Unroll and separate crescent roll dough into triangles. Wrap each piece of apple in a crescent roll. Arrange in a greased 8"x8" baking pan; sprinkle with cinnamon. Combine butter, sugar and orange juice in a medium saucepan. Bring to a boil; remove from heat and stir in vanilla. Pour mixture over dumplings; sprinkle pecans over top. Bake at 350 degrees for 30 minutes, or until crust is golden and beginning to bubble. To serve, spoon some of the syrup from the baking pan over dumplings. Serve with ice cream, if desired.

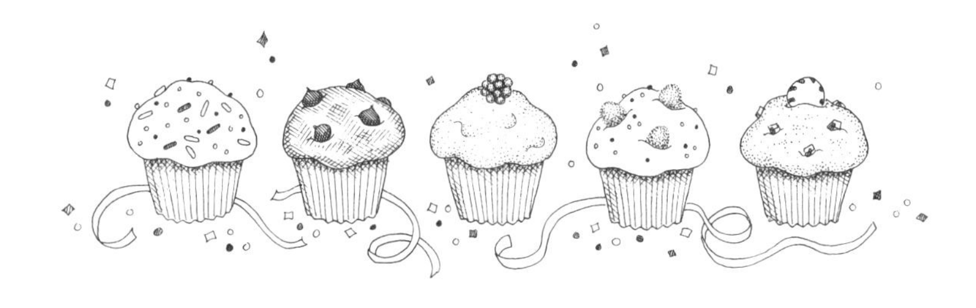

Bake up some tie-dyed cupcakes...it's simple! Just prepare a yellow cake mix as directed, then divide the batter among three bowls and tint each one a different color. Scoop equal amounts of batter into each cupcake liner and swirl gently with a knife. Bake as directed.

## Dirt Cups

*Makes 4 servings*

- 2 c. milk
- 3.9-oz. pkg. instant chocolate pudding mix
- 8-oz. container frozen whipped topping, thawed
- 16-oz. pkg. chocolate sandwich cookies, crushed and divided
- 4 9-oz. clear plastic cups
- Garnish: gummi worms, gummi frogs, peanuts and granola

Whisk milk and pudding mix together until well blended; let stand for 5 minutes. Fold in whipped topping and half the crushed cookies; set aside. Spoon one tablespoon remaining crushed cookies into each cup; fill 3/4 full with pudding. Sprinkle with remaining crushed cookies; refrigerate at least one hour or until ready to serve. Garnish with gummi creatures, peanut "rocks" and granola "sand."

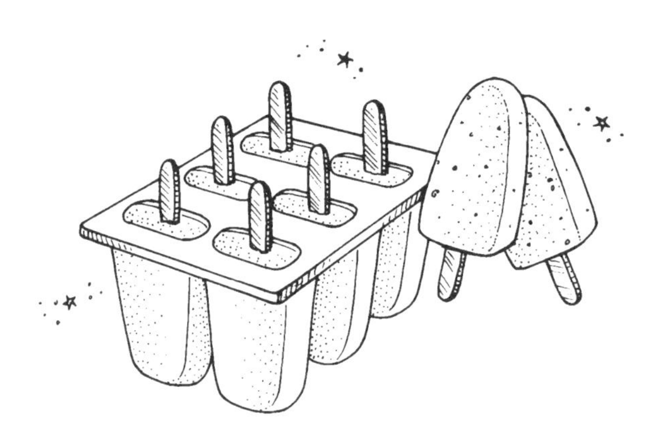

Yummy yogurt bars! Blend 8 ounces of plain yogurt with
8 to 10 ounces of peeled and chopped fresh fruit. Strawberries,
bananas and peaches are especially yummy. Blend yogurt for
15 seconds in a blender; add fruit and blend until smooth. Pour into
popsicle molds and freeze. Makes six cool and creamy bars.

## Giant Cookie

*Serves 12*

2-1/4 c. all-purpose flour
1 t. baking powder
1/2 t. salt
1 c. butter, softened
1-1/2 c. brown sugar, packed
1 t. vanilla extract
2 eggs
2 c. milk chocolate chips
16-oz. container chocolate frosting
Garnish: milk chocolate chunks, mini marshmallows, peanuts

In a small bowl, combine flour, baking powder and salt; set aside. Use an electric mixer on medium speed to beat together butter, brown sugar and vanilla for 5 minutes. Add eggs, one at a time, beating well after each addition. Gradually beat in flour mixture; stir in chocolate chips. Spread batter on a 14" round pizza pan lined with parchment paper. Bake at 375 degrees for 30 to 40 minutes, until golden. Cool in pan for 10 minutes. Transfer to a serving platter to cool completely. Decorate as desired with chocolate frosting; sprinkle edges with garnishes. To serve, cut into wedges.

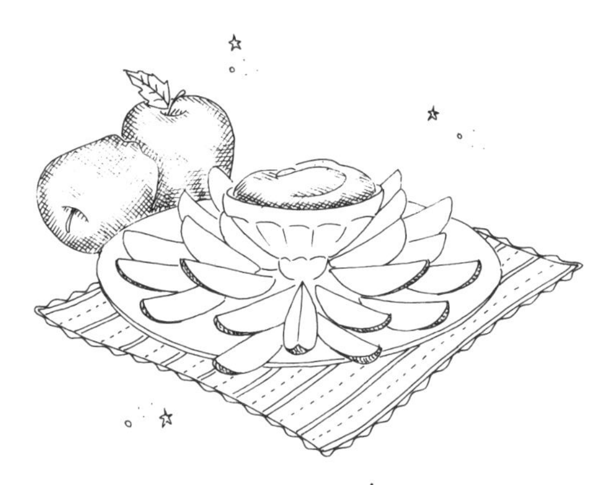

Homemade caramel apple dip...yum! Spray a slow cooker with non-stick vegetable spray and pour in two cans of sweetened condensed milk. Cover and cook on low setting for 2-1/2 hours, until milk thickens; stir. Replace lid and continue cooking another one to 1-1/2 hours, stirring every 15 minutes, until thick and golden. Serve warm or chilled; store in the refrigerator.

## *Ice Cream Sandwich Cake*

*Makes 12 servings*

12 ice cream sandwiches
8-oz. container frozen whipped topping, thawed
12-oz. jar chocolate ice cream topping
Garnish: candy sprinkles, crushed candy bars, crushed cookies

Arrange ice cream sandwiches to fit in a 13"x9" baking pan, using as many as needed and cutting some in half if necessary. Spread with whipped topping; drizzle with chocolate topping. Sprinkle desired garnishes over the top. Cover pan and freeze for about one hour, until whipped topping is firm. At serving time, cut into slices.

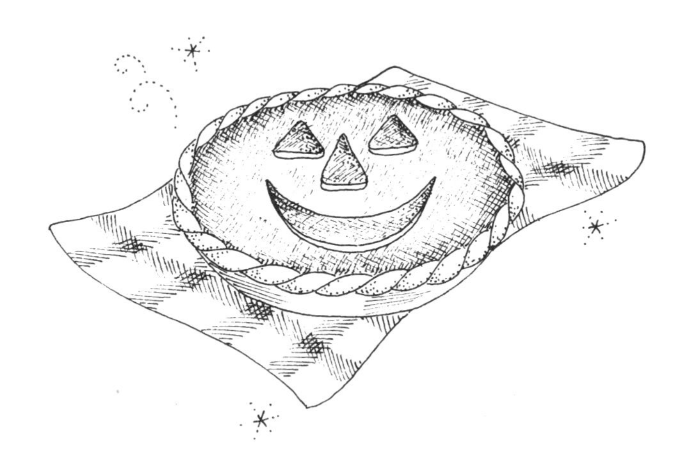

Dress up Honey-Pumpkin Pie with a smile! Roll out remaining pie crust dough and cut out three triangles...two for eyes, one for a nose. Place them on an unbaked pie. Add a smile with a crescent moon-shaped portion of dough; bake as directed.

## *Honey-Pumpkin Pie*

*Makes 6 to 8 servings*

15-oz. can pumpkin
3/4 c. honey
1/2 t. salt
1 t. cinnamon
1/2 t. ground ginger
1/4 t. ground cloves
1/4 t. nutmeg
3 eggs, beaten
2/3 c. evaporated milk
1/2 c. milk
9-inch pie crust

Stir together pumpkin, honey, salt and spices in a large mixing bowl. Add eggs and mix well; stir in milks. Place pie crust in a 9" pie plate; flute edges forming a high rim to hold pumpkin mixture. Do not pierce crust. Pour in pumpkin mixture. Bake at 375 degrees for 55 to 60 minutes, until set. Let cool before serving.

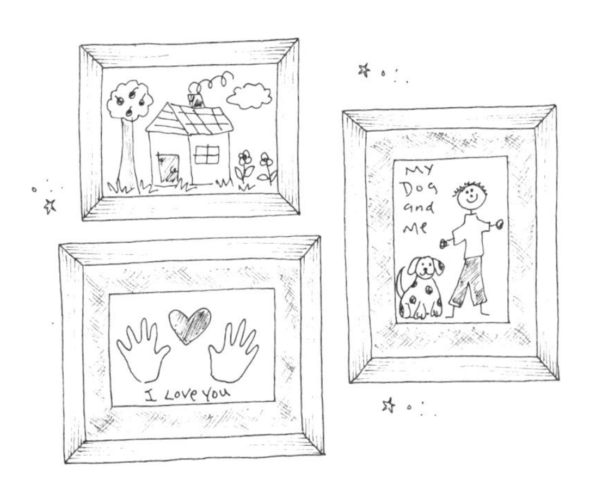


Are the refrigerator doors overwhelmed with crayon masterpieces? Select a few special drawings to have matted and framed...the kids will be so proud!

## Triple Fudgy Brownies

*Makes about 1-1/2 dozen*

3.4-oz. pkg. instant chocolate pudding mix
2 c. milk
18-1/2 oz. pkg. chocolate cake mix
Optional: 1 t. vanilla or almond extract
12-oz. pkg. semi-sweet chocolate chips
Optional: powdered sugar

Combine dry pudding mix and milk; stir just until pudding starts to thicken. Stir in dry cake mix and extract, if using. Fold in chocolate chips. Spread batter evenly into a lightly greased 13"x9" baking pan; place on center oven rack. Bake at 350 degrees for about 30 to 40 minutes, until top springs back when lightly touched. Let cool at least one hour before cutting into squares. Dust with powdered sugar, if desired.

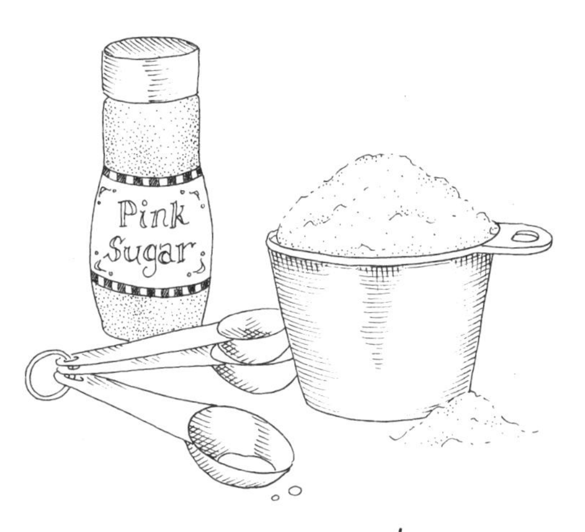


Make your own colored sugar...easy! Place a cup of sugar in a plastic zipping bag, then add two or three drops of food coloring. Knead the bag until color is mixed throughout, then spread sugar on a baking sheet to dry.

## Powerballs

*Makes about 3-1/2 dozen*

1 c. creamy peanut butter
1 c. honey
3 c. long-cooking oats, uncooked
1/2 c. ground flaxseed
1 c. semi-sweet chocolate chips
1/2 c. dry-roasted peanuts, coarsely chopped
1/4 c. raisins
1/4 c. sweetened dried cranberries

In a large bowl, mix together peanut butter and honey until smooth. Gradually add oats and flaxseed; mix well. Fold in chocolate chips, peanuts and dried fruit; blend together gently. Roll into one-inch balls and place on lightly greased baking sheets. Cover and refrigerate overnight.

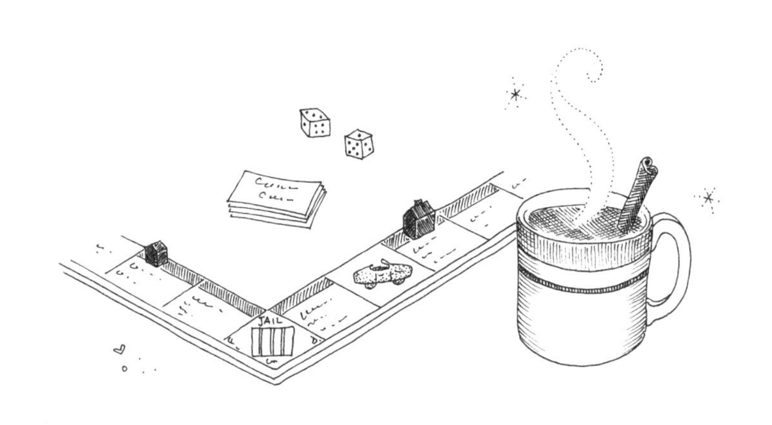


Hot chocolate is a great bedtime beverage...the warm milk acts as a sleep inducer.

## Slumber Party Pizza

*Makes 8 to 10 servings*

18-oz. tube refrigerated peanut butter cookie dough
1-1/2 c. semi-sweet chocolate chips
2 c. mini marshmallows
12-oz. jar caramel ice cream topping

Roll out cookie dough onto a 12" pizza pan; bake for 7 minutes according to package directions. Remove from oven; immediately sprinkle the top with chocolate chips and marshmallows. Drizzle with caramel topping. Bake for another 5 minutes, or until chocolate chips begin to melt. Cool for 5 to 10 minutes. Cut into wedges to serve.

# INDEX

# INDEX

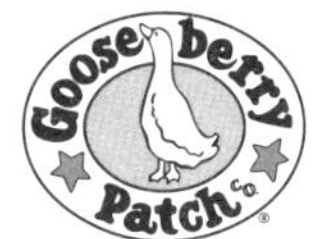


# Our Story

Back in 1984, we were next-door neighbors raising our families in the little town of Delaware, Ohio. Two moms with small children, we were looking for a way to do what we loved and stay home with the kids too. We had always shared a love of home cooking and making memories with family & friends and so, after many a conversation over the backyard fence, **Gooseberry Patch** was born.

We put together our first catalog at our kitchen tables, enlisting the help of our loved ones wherever we could. From that very first mailing, we found an immediate connection with many of our customers and it wasn't long before we began receiving letters, photos and recipes from these new friends. In 1992, we put together our very first cookbook, compiled from hundreds of these recipes and, the rest, as they say, is history.

Hard to believe it's been over 25 years since those kitchen-table days! From that original little **Gooseberry Patch** family, we've grown to include an amazing group of creative folks who love cooking, decorating and creating as much as we do. Today, we're best known for our homestyle, family-friendly cookbooks, now recognized as national bestsellers.

One thing's for sure, we couldn't have done it without our friends all across the country. Each year, we're honored to turn thousands of your recipes into our collectible cookbooks. Our hope is that each book captures the stories and heart of all of you who have shared with us. Whether you've been with us since the beginning or are just discovering us, welcome to the **Gooseberry Patch** family!

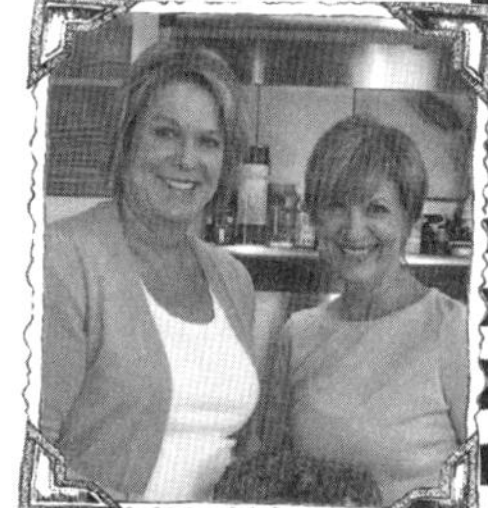

*JoAnn & Vickie*

Visit our website anytime

**www.gooseberrypatch.com**

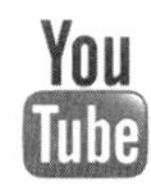

1·800·854·6673